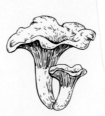

HOW TO FORAGE FOR MUSHROOMS
without dying

AN ABSOLUTE BEGINNER'S GUIDE
to identifying 29 wild, edible mushrooms

FRANK HYMAN

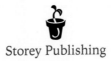

Storey Publishing

The mission of Storey Publishing is to serve our customers by
publishing practical information that encourages
personal independence in harmony with the environment.

Edited by Carleen Madigan
Art direction and book design by
   Carolyn Eckert and Stacy Wakefield Forte
Text production by Stacy Wakefield Forte
   and Jennifer Jepson Smith
Indexed by Samantha Miller

Cover photography by © Barbora Batokova/
   stock.adobe.com, bk. row 4 r.; © Evgenij
   Yulkin/Stocksy, bk. inside; © frolova_elena/
   stock.adobe.com, bk. row 2 r.; © Ionescu
   Bogdan/stock.adobe.com, bk. row 1 l.;
   © JohnatAPW/stock.adobe.com, bk.
   row 4 l.; Krzysztof Niewolny/Unsplash,
   front; Lebrac/Wikimedia Commons/CC
   BY-SA 3.0, bk. row 3 r.; © Lisa Mackie/
   Shutterstock.com, bk. row 1 r.; © Liz
   Nemeth, bk. au.; © misuma/iStock.com,
   frt. inside; © Pihuliak/stock.adobe.com, bk.
   row 3 l.; © PiLensPhoto/stock.adobe.com,
   bk. row 5 l.; © Ramona Heim/stock.adobe
   .com, bk. row 2 l.; © valeriyap/stock.adobe
   .com, bk. row 5 r.
**Interior photography credits appear
   on page 254**

Text © 2021 by Frank Hyman

Storey Publishing
210 MASS MoCA Way
North Adams, MA 01247
storey.com

Storey Publishing, LLC is an imprint of
Workman Publishing Co., Inc., a subsidiary of
Hachette Book Group, Inc., 1290 Avenue of
the Americas, New York, NY 10104

Printed in China by R.R. Donnelley
10 9 8 7 6 5

ISBNs: 978-1-63586-332-1 (paper);
   978-1-63586-333-8 (ebook)

Library of Congress Cataloging-in-
   Publication Data on file

Storey books are available at special discounts when purchased in bulk for premiums
and sales promotions as well as for fund-raising or educational use. Special editions or book
excerpts can also be created to specification. For details, please email to
special.markets@hbgusa.com.

HOW TO
FORAGE FOR MUSHROOMS
without dying

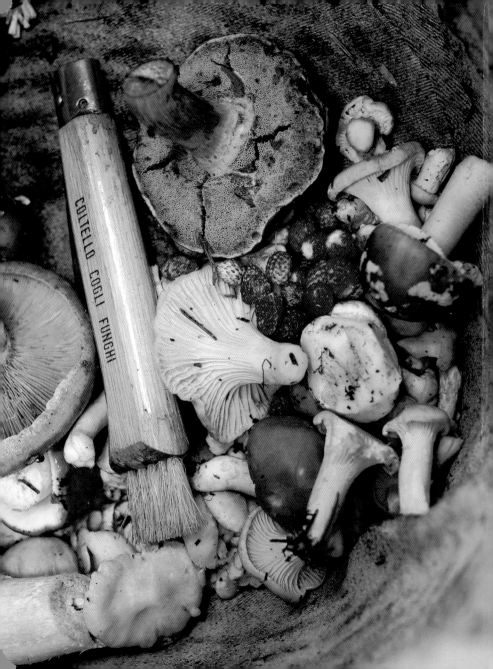

This book is dedicated to the memory of Beatrix Potter,
a forager and feminist ahead of her time.

And to my niece, fellow forager,
and favorite wood sprite, Avery Crochetière,
whom I know to be fully capable
of picking up Potter's torch and carrying on.

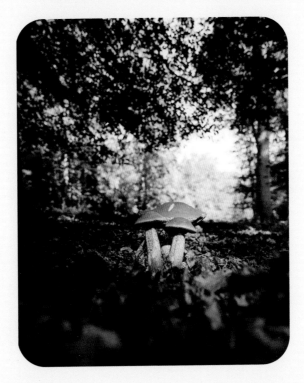

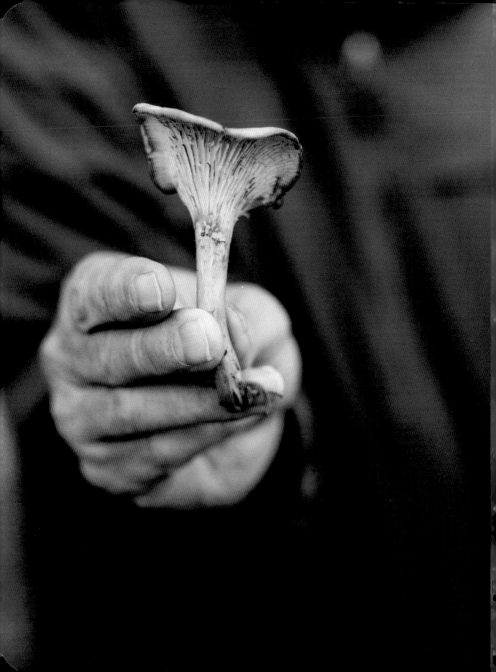

Contents

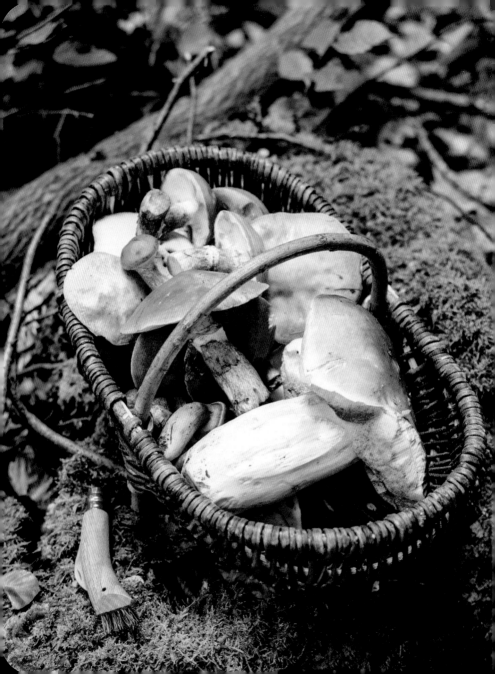

What's Different about This Book?

This book is not like other mushroom ID books. But that doesn't mean there's anything wrong with it. Actually, this is the book that I wish I'd had when I first started foraging.

- It's compact.

- It only covers common mushrooms that you'll want to eat, use, or avoid.

- The descriptions focus on important details that differentiate each mushroom from its look-alikes.

- Latin names are translated.

- It omits subjective mushroom characteristics that aren't critical, that vary in the field, and that are subjective, like aroma.

- The mushrooms aren't arranged alphabetically (novices don't know their names yet!) but by what the novice forager does know: the season, the mushrooms' location (on wood or on the ground), and whether or not they have gills.

- Almost all the mushrooms in this book can be safely identified in the field without knowing the spore print color. I've still included the spore print color in the What, Where & When sections, for your own knowledge.

- It provides a few stories for the sake of sharing the flavor of what it's like to be a forager.

- It contains links to professional foragers' recipes (see page 242) and techniques for preparing and storing fungi (see page 211).

- And it has a sense of humor. I hope.

Another thing that's different about this book is that it's written by a mushroom hunter for other mushroom hunters. I've been foraging since 2004. I've learned my trade from foragers in eight US states and six countries, and I'm certified to safely sell wild mushrooms to the public in three US states. But I don't have a degree in mycology (the branch of biology dealing with fungi). Most of the tens of millions of people who successfully forage wild mushrooms on this planet don't have a degree in mycology. And to safely hunt edible mushrooms, you don't need one either.

WHAT'S FOR DINNER?

Throughout the book, we've included the following icons to serve as quick indicators of whether or not a mushroom can be safely eaten. Be sure also to read the text that accompanies the mushroom in question, in case there are additional factors to consider.

An edible species

A medicinal species

A species you should not eat,
either because it could make you sick,
its edibility is unknown,
or it just doesn't taste good

A species that could kill you
if you eat it

WHAT THOSE OTHER BOOKS HAVE

Many, if not most, mushroom ID books are written by degreed mycologists to appeal to other degreed mycologists and very serious hobbyists. And that's all well and good. Truly. For intermediate and advanced mushroom hunters, that can be useful. I own and enjoy many of those books myself. But some—not all—of those books have tendencies that aren't always helpful to the novice and intermediate mushroom hunter:

- They frequently use Latin terminology in places where plain English would suffice.

- When Latin names are given, the species names aren't translated.

- Many descriptions include details that don't help separate the wheat from the chaff, so to speak.

- Many descriptions leave out salient identification details that would differentiate an unappealing or poisonous look-alike.

- They read like a textbook. Which they are. Which is fine. But that's not necessarily the best format for every beginner.

There are many books written by mycologists that I can recommend for those ready to attain intermediate or expert status (see page 240). Consider this compact volume your Foraging 101 book. If you want to go further, pick up some more books.

Meanwhile, stash this book in your back pocket, glove box, purse, or bag and get outside where the mushrooms are. You can't eat 'em if you don't find 'em. And you can't find 'em if you're not outside. I know that's where I'll be.

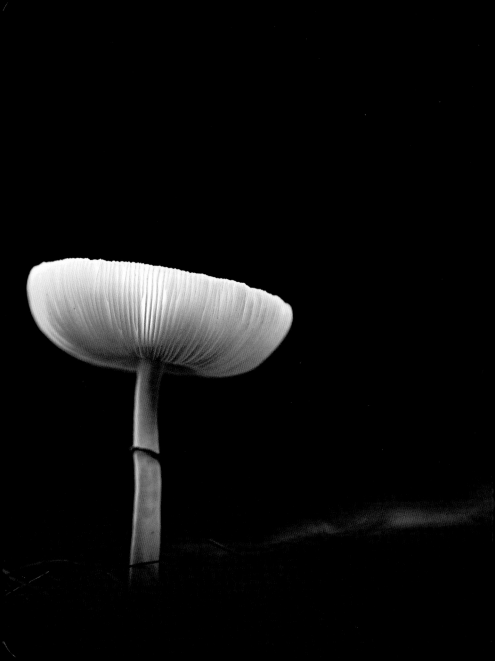

CHAPTER 1

WHAT THE HECK ARE MUSHROOMS,
Anyway?

There are many thousands of species of fungi.
But we're only interested in a handful of them:
those with visible fruiting parts that
might be edible, medicinal, or poisonous.
These fruiting parts are what the average person
typically calls "a mushroom."

WHERE DID MUSHROOMS COME FROM?

If you crammed the 4.5-billion-year history of the Earth into one 24-hour day, the birth of Earth would start at midnight. At that point, there's only bare rock, meteorites, and thunderstorms. Rain rubs the stones into clay, silt, and sand particles that cook up thick, minerally, muddy stews and watery, salty soups.

Finally after a half-billion years of these random molecules mixing, some of them click together like a Rubik's Cube to become the first living things: one-celled microbes. It's 4 a.m. For another half-billion or so years these microbes evolve into a variety of one-celled creatures to match conditions on Earth. Or maybe it should be called Ocean. That is what covers most of the surface and is where all the life-forms can be found partying at this point. It finally occurs to these microbes to start leaving graffiti in the form of fossils around 6 a.m.

A couple billion years later, single-celled algae show up and invent photosynthesis. It's around 2 p.m. The pace picks up. Sort of. Things move along swimmingly at sea with the arrival of jellyfish just before 9 p.m. We've been waiting for forests for about 4 billion years now. Land plants show up just before 10 p.m. Giant ferns' living bodies come into being by combining (1) a Goodyear Blimp–worth of carbon dioxide, (2) busloads of liquid water, and (3) some loose pocket change of minerals. But plants, and eventually trees, die, fall to the ground, and pile up into vast untapped bank accounts of nutrients. Unable to decompose properly, those prefungal jungles—composed mostly of carbon—compress into coal and oil.

By 11 p.m. some of the microbes evolve into simple fungi with a special hunger. They attack these sheaves of dead jungle matter and suck the marrow of energy from them. Without these fungi,

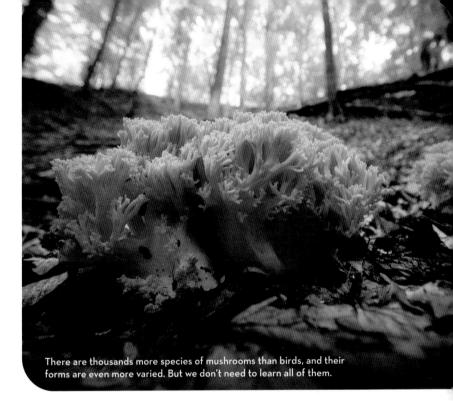

There are thousands more species of mushrooms than birds, and their forms are even more varied. But we don't need to learn all of them.

we'd be neck deep in the dead plants of the last half-billion years. That or swimming in oil. A few other fungi species go full-on gangster and assassinate trees to make their living. A third group of fungi choose to go underground to become the nursing mothers of teeming forests.

At 11:59 p.m. humans find themselves in a thick Eden and they're hungry. They discover the mysterious fungi. They learn from trial and error. And just as not everything that glitters is gold, they learn that not everything that tastes or smells good is food. Which brings us to right now, with you reading this book.

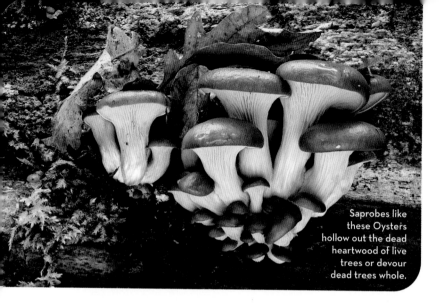

Saprobes like these Oysters hollow out the dead heartwood of live trees or devour dead trees whole.

WHAT IS THEIR M.O.
(MODUS OPERANDI)?

Knowing how and why mushrooms do what they do helps the novice mushroom detective discover the secret identities of these mysterious creatures.

EATERS OF THE DEAD: SAPROBES

The fungi that devour dead plant and animal matter are called saprobes or saprophytes. Some of the mushrooms growing on the ground are saprobes, breaking down organic matter of grasses (such as Puffballs) or dropped branches on or in the ground (such as Devil's Urn). Many of the mushrooms that grow on tree trunks are also saprobes (such as Lion's Mane), which are eating the dead wood of downed trees or the dead heartwood of standing trees with a still-living sapwood. The most common cultivated mushrooms are saprobes: Oysters, Shiitake, Hen of the Woods, and others.

As you may remember from middle-school biology, the cells under a tree's bark are alive and called the cambium and the sapwood. Those layers are composed of vertical tubes that send water and nutrients up from the roots and parallel tubes that bring down sugar created by the photosynthetic leaves.

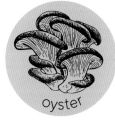

oyster

The oldest cells at the center of the tree form what's called the heartwood. These cells have died from old age and are empty (that's where the saprophytic fungi might be found on a live tree). The living cells are producing waste material, which has to go somewhere. So horizontal tubes carry that waste from the living cells to store it in the empty, dead, heartwood cells. So when you smell the fragrance of the heartwood of cedar, you are actually sniffing tree poop (think about that next time you stick your head into a cedar-lined closet).

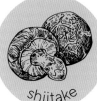

shiitake

Cedar tree poop is so strong that most fungi don't like to eat it. That's why cedar trees are used for fence posts; they resist fungal rot. But the heartwood of other trees doesn't do such a great job of fending off fungi. So when you find a hollow tree, what you're seeing is the heartwood that has been eaten by saprophytic fungi. Which begs the question, "What is the sapwood doing with all its waste products if it can't dump them in the heartwood anymore?" I have a theory, but that is clearly beyond the scope of this book! Ask a tree surgeon!

EATERS OF THE LIVING: PARASITES

A much smaller number of fungi species attack living wood and eat those cells. These types of fungi are called parasites, a term from medieval French meaning a person who eats from the table of another. Ringed Honey Mushrooms are one example.

A tree being consumed by a saprobe can live indefinitely, since it's only losing its dead cells. But a tree infected by a parasite like a Honey Mushroom has an expiration date. One easy sign that a mature tree is in poor health, possibly from a fungal parasite, is bare twigs and branches at the outer edge of the canopy.

If you want to try to help such a tree on your property, you will find people happy to sell you fungicidal products, but these don't actually kill any fungus. They simply inhibit its reproduction a bit and have to be used for a long time. A. Long. Time. And even then, the likelihood of success is low.

When a tree (or a garden plant) is stricken by a fungus on its leaves, that's often a temporary problem that can be diminished, if not resolved, by moving the plant (if small enough) to a place with more sunlight and better air movement. Or by spraying diluted milk on the leaves periodically (yes, really). But when a parasitic fungus is in the roots or in the trunk, the game is up. However, that doesn't mean you necessarily have an emergency. It helps to think of trees as living and dying in slow motion compared to animals.

If the infected tree can fall on a house, get some estimates for removal and then start saving up. Or move. Or at least keep your insurance paid up. And then when you see Honey Mushrooms nearby, whether you eat them or not, bag them up for the trash ASAP to minimize the spread of their spores.

MARRIED MUSHROOMS: MYCORRHIZAL

The third type of fungi connects and collaborates with the roots of trees. These are called mycorrhizal. The term "myco" means fungus. The term "rhyza" refers to the roots of plants.

As in any good marriage, each participant provides what it does well. Trees share the sugars they make from photosynthesis in the

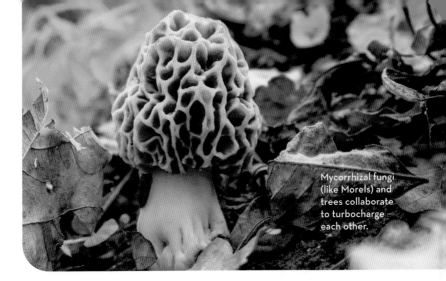
Mycorrhizal fungi (like Morels) and trees collaborate to turbocharge each other.

leaves. Fungi share surplus moisture and nutrients that they are better able to extract from the soil.

And as in human marriages, there are variations in practices and in degree of mutuality between mycorrhizal fungi and their woody partners. Those details are not necessary to learn mushroom ID, but what is good to know is that learning tree species can help a forager find mycorrhizal mushrooms like Morels. They grow in the company of elms, ashes, tulip poplars, cottonwoods, and apple trees. Who knows what those tree species have in common that suits Morels? But if none of those are around, then you certainly won't find Morels. Other mycorrhizal fungi like Chanterelles are more promiscuous. They might shack up with a wide variety of deciduous trees or evergreens.

morels

One last thing that's helpful to know is that cultivating mycorrhizal mushrooms is even more difficult than successfully arranging a human marriage between strangers. In fact, no one that I'm aware of has managed it.

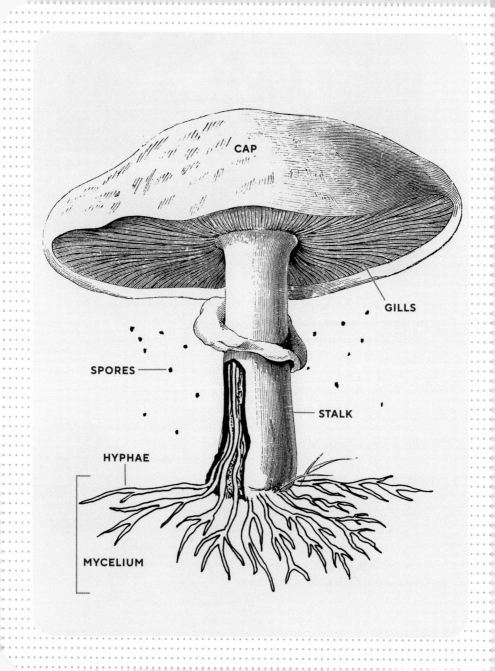

FUNGAL ANATOMY

In many mushroom ID books, this can be one of the least fun parts for novices to pick up. Especially if you struggled in science classes. So, to help you get off the ground in your education on mushrooms, I'm going to strip down and simplify things in a way that some mycologists may not like. You don't have to know the names of every part of a mushroom or every phase of its growth to be a successful mushroom hunter. That's why I'll just be addressing those things that answer basic questions and help with identification. But you'll have a great grounding in how mushrooms do their work and play their roles because I'm going to explain them in terms of things you already have some familiarity with: plants and animals.

HOW ARE THEY LIKE PLANTS?

Mushrooms have a number of different parts that help them collect necessary nutrients, grow, and reproduce. In order to understand how these different parts work, it's useful to think of them in terms of their plant analogues: roots, trunk and branches, fruits, and seeds.

ROOTS: HYPHAE

What would be called roots in a plant are called hyphae in a mushroom. In all the fungi in this book, the hyphae are doing work similar to plant roots: extracting moisture and nutrients. In mycorrhizal fungi, the hyphae connect and collaborate with their counterparts (tree roots) to acquire sugar. Those connected hyphae are bartering for the sugar with nutrients and moisture gathered by other hyphae. In saprobes and parasites, hyphae devour cells, either dead (saprobes) or living (parasites), to gather energy, moisture, and nutrients.

TRUNK AND BRANCHES: MYCELIUM

A mushroom's mycelium can be thought of as functioning like the growing, spreading trunk and branches of a tree. Mycologists consider mycelium to be the vegetative part of the fungus. Mycelia are composed of hyphae. If you've ever broken off some bark and seen a sticky, thready, white network of fungus underneath, that's mostly mycelium with hyphae forming the outer threads. The term "mycelium" derives from the Greek word for fungus: *mýkitas*.

FRUIT: THE MUSHROOM ITSELF

If, and only if, the fungi have the right amount of nutrients, energy, and moisture and if the season and temperature are just right, then they will send out the edible mushrooms that we seek. This is called fruiting. Whether we're talking about a fungal shelf on a tree or a stalk and cap coming out of the ground, the mushrooms described in this book are considered fruits. And even though not all fungal fruits are edible, they still function much like the fruit of a tree.

One important difference is that plants like to flower and set fruit on a pretty reliable timeline that reflects day length and soil temperature. Even in suboptimal conditions, plants produce some kind of fruit on a predictable schedule. Fungi, on the other hand, will take the year off or come earlier or later depending on environmental conditions. For me, a recent drought in the months of August and September caused Hen of the Woods to skip a year entirely.

Sometimes the speed with which fungal fruit grows shocks people. Many times, the fruits "mushroom" to full size overnight. The explanation for that speed is that before the fruit comes forth, the fungus has created all of the fruit's cells, but in miniature. When ready, the mycelium fills those tiny cells with water, and they inflate like a balloon to a mature size in a matter of hours or days.

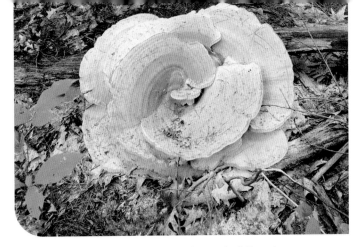

The fruit of the fungus (often called the "fruiting body") produces spores. Sometimes you can see the spores coloring their surroundings.

The initial stage of growth is called the pin. When it's very young and fresh it's called a button. When mature it's called the fruit.

SEEDS: SPORES

Tree fruits are a delivery mechanism for getting seeds out into the world to produce the next generation. Likewise, fungal fruits are a way to get spores out into the world to produce the next generation. Spores are the dusty specks that drop out of gills, false gills, pores, and other structures. Their large numbers are an indication that only a small percentage of spores are expected to be successful.

Spores function like seeds in several ways. Many of them expect to be blown on the wind to new territory. But the infamous Stinkhorn smells like dog poop for a reason. Flies are attracted to it, and after saying "I coulda swore I smelled some dog poop over here," they fly away disappointed yet covered in Stinkhorn spores—much like a bee covered in pollen.

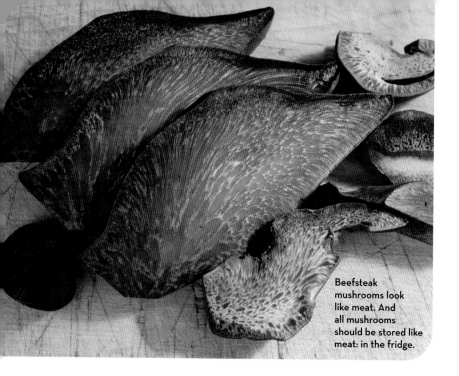

Beefsteak mushrooms look like meat. And all mushrooms should be stored like meat: in the fridge.

HOW ARE THEY LIKE ANIMALS?

The fruits of edible mushrooms are partly made of chitin. In animals, chitin forms the shells of insects and crustaceans. (A similar material, keratin, forms hair, fur, claws, and nails on other animals.) Humans can't digest chitin in mushrooms without cooking it—one of several reasons it's best to cook edible mushrooms before eating them.

Another important similarity between animals and edible mushrooms is that, like animal meat, edible mushrooms must be handled and stored with care. You can leave vegetables unrefrigerated overnight and they may get a little older, but they rarely go bad. If mushrooms are left at room temperature overnight or in the back

Mushrooms left unrefrigerated can make you as sick as raw meat left on the counter overnight.

seat of a hot car all afternoon, they will likely grow a nasty layer of bacteria on their surface, as meat would. Many cases of sickness attributed to mushrooms are actually instances of correctly identified edible mushrooms that have been poorly handled and caused food poisoning. It's just as if you'd left raw hamburger on the counter overnight before cooking it.

Always store edible mushrooms (whether wild or store-bought) in paper bags rather than plastic (see page 213 for more on why) and toss them in the fridge or on ice as soon as you can.

CAPS OR CUPS?
WHAT'S THAT PART CALLED?

I love me some plain English. But I also have a degree in horticulture, so I've learned a lot of Latin names for plants and the fungi that plague them. And if I were a mycologist and I were talking to another mycologist, you would hear the Latin names fly. But I'm just a lowly mushroom hunter (although one certified to sell wild mushrooms in three US states). And likely as not, you're a wannabe mushroom hunter (or perhaps a shaky intermediate mushroom hunter or even an expert mushroom hunter, yet suffering from "imposter syndrome"). So learning to identify mushrooms is plenty of responsibility without having to learn Latin, too. Although, if you get more serious about foraging and acquire other books, you probably will pick up some of the lingo. (Fun fact: "Lingo" derives from the Latin word *lingua*, meaning language.) For now, I'm going to use some plain English in describing the various parts of a mushroom. Here we go.

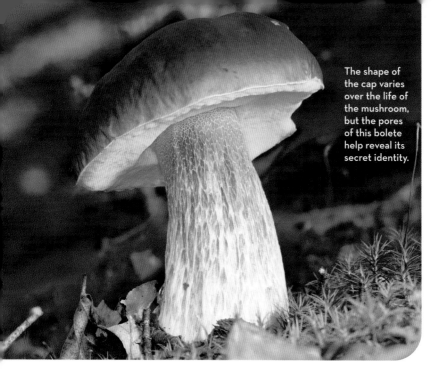

The shape of the cap varies over the life of the mushroom, but the pores of this bolete help reveal its secret identity.

CAP

In the everyday image of a mushroom, it grows from the ground on a vertical stalk and has a horizontal cap. When the mushroom first pops up from the soil, the cap is hugging the stalk like a closed umbrella. Then it flares out like an open umbrella. Many times, the cap of an older mushroom will flex upward like a blown-out umbrella. All mushrooms with caps go through these stages, so they are not useful in differentiating edible mushrooms from their look-alikes. That's why you won't see me mentioning this phenomenon in the ID portion of this book. On the other hand, the size, color, and texture of the upper side and lower sides of the cap often help determine a mushroom's secret identity.

GILLS OR PORES

Look under the cap and you will find either deep, parallel gills or spongelike pores. Both structures are for releasing spores. With some species, the gills or pores may start out as one color and change to another color. This is caused by the color of the spores. Finding a patch of mixed-aged mushrooms that are clearly the same species but have different colored gills or pores can help determine the ID. Damaging some gills or pores may cause a stain to show up, and this can also help with ID. Other damaged gills may release what looks like milk, which means you have a mushroom from the genus *Lactarius*. In Latin, *lac* means "milk."

A spongy layer beneath the cap indicates the pores of a bolete, if the mushroom is growing from a stalk on the ground. If the spongy layer is on a shelf or bracket (see page 30) growing from a tree, it's likely a polypore (which simply means "many pores") like Chicken of the Woods or Reishi. The pore layers look similar, and both surfaces serve the same purpose of dispensing spores.

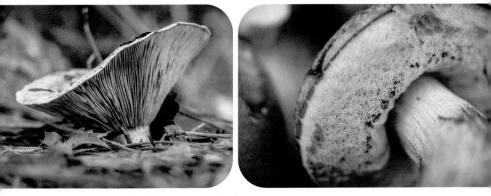

Break some gills; if they release milk, it's a *Lactarius* species.
Right: Squeeze pores on boletes to see if they change color.

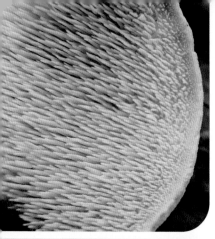

TEETH OR SPINES

Spines may cover the underside of the cap of mushrooms that grow on the ground, such as Hedgehogs. Or they may cover almost the entire mushroom, as with Lion's Mane. Whatever you call them—teeth or spines—they serve the same purpose: to disperse spores.

FALSE GILLS

Under the caps of some mushrooms, you may find what look like gills but are considered to be false gills. Chanterelles are a great example of this feature. Look closely: What you're seeing are less like deep, parallel gills and more like shallow ridges that make forks and crosses (or Vs, Xs, and Ys). They perform the same function as true gills and are a boon to novice mushroom hunters, because they will help you sort edible Chanterelles from Sickeners like Jack O'Lanterns.

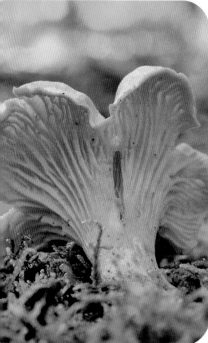

You might have an edible mushroom if you find teeth or false gills under the cap.

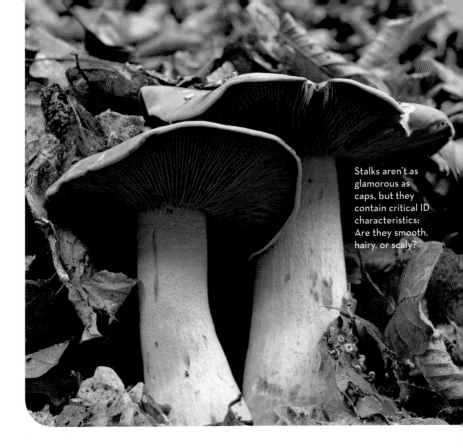

Stalks aren't as glamorous as caps, but they contain critical ID characteristics: Are they smooth, hairy, or scaly?

STALK

Most caps come with a stalk, also called a stem. It's the central pillar that holds up the cap. If it's coming out of a tree, it might be off-center under the cap. It may be so short as to not be obvious. It sometimes helps to cut the stalk open to see if it is a different color than the skin and to see if it stains once exposed to air or pressure. Some mushrooms may have little or no stalk at all. If the stalk snaps like a piece of chalk, it is either a Russula or Milk Cap.

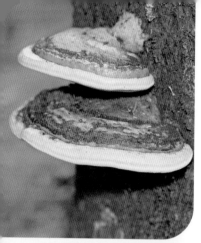

SHELF OR BRACKET

Some mushrooms that grow from trees have a horizontal cap that has little or no stalk. Artist's Conk is an example of this growth form. The term "shelf" is used if the mushroom is mostly flat like a pizza. The term "bracket" is more often used if they have a not-so-flat shape like Tinder Conk.

SPORES

When spores drop from a mushroom, they will discolor the gills or pores. This can be an important ID clue for some mushrooms. If there are overlapping layers of mushrooms in a clump, the spore color may show up on top of the caps of lower mushrooms. If there's no indication of the spore color, you can take a cap home and put it on a piece of newspaper overnight to leave a spore print. Dark-colored spores will show up on the light-colored part of the paper and even white spores will show up covering the printed part of the newspaper. Fortunately, almost every mushroom I've chosen for this book can be identified in the field, without waiting to see the spore color.

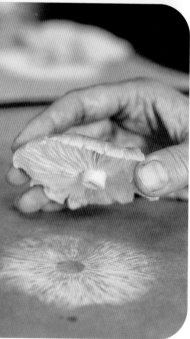

The color of a mushroom's spores can help identify the species.

Is it a Puffball? Cut it open to find out: it should be solid white inside.

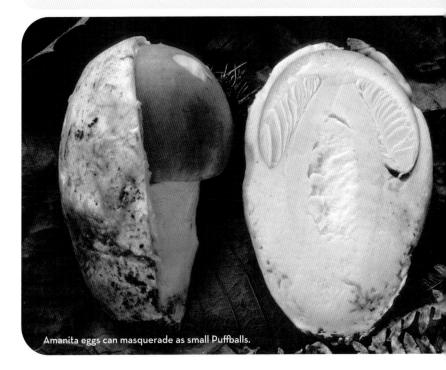

Amanita eggs can masquerade as small Puffballs.

EGG

Amanitas hatch from eggs that are found in the soil. Some might mistake them for dirty Puffballs. But cutting one open reveals the outline of a cartoon mushroom. Or if it's a Stinkhorn egg, it will reveal a gelatinous space alien. As the mushroom inflates and breaks the egg apart, it may leave warts or a partial veil on the cap and/or a ring or skirt (I like to call it a tutu) around the stalk. The egg will always leave a cup or fat collar at the base of the stalk.

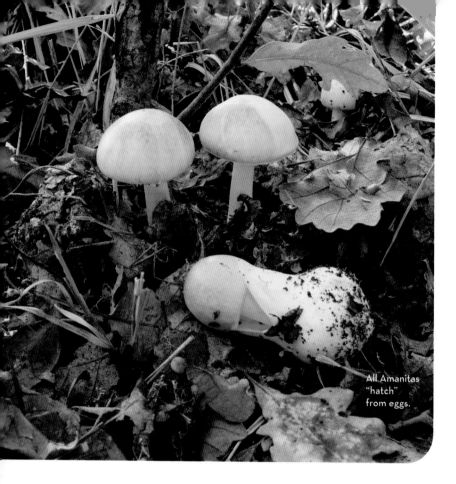

All Amanitas "hatch" from eggs.

CUP

The wise novice digs up the base of all unfamiliar mushrooms, because the dirty base of the stalk may be erupting from a cup or a thick collar. Both are signs of potentially poisonous mushrooms. The cup or collar is the bottom portion of the egg that some mushrooms hatch from.

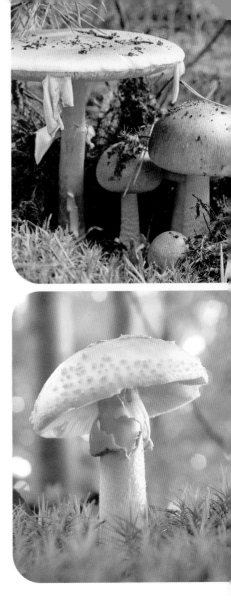

VEIL

The top and middle portions of the egg are called the veil—another sign of a potentially poisonous mushroom. The top portion of the veil may leave shredded bits on top of the cap or a damaged sheet that covers part of the cap, or may disappear altogether in the rain.

WARTS

This is another term for the shredded bits of the egg or veil left on top of the cap.

RING

The middle portion of the veil covers the gills until the expanding mushroom tears it apart. There may be little of the middle portion of the veil to see, so look carefully. Often the middle portion of the veil will leave a ring/skirt/tutu around the stalk. But sometimes this will fall off or just leave a stain on the stalk.

After the cap shreds its veil (top), a ring is left around the stalk (bottom).

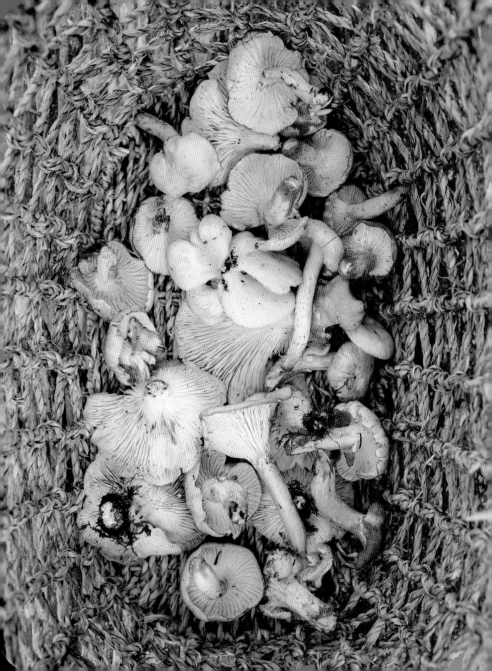

CHAPTER 2

SAFE & RESPONSIBLE *Foraging*

Millions of mushroom hunters around the world forage safely, and you can, too. The best way to avoid getting sick is to learn how to identify mushrooms accurately, handle them properly after harvesting, cook them well, and don't eat too much of them on the first go-round. Always exercise good judgment, be cautious, and if you're not 100 percent sure of a mushroom's identity, do not eat it!

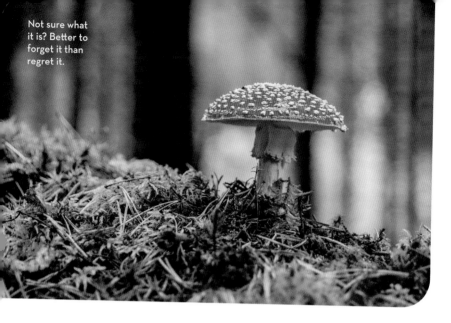

Not sure what it is? Better to forget it than regret it.

HOW NOT TO GET SICK OR DIE FROM EATING WILD MUSHROOMS

There are two foolproof ways to avoid getting poisoned by mushrooms. The first way is to never, ever eat a mushroom. But how much fun is that?

The second way—and to my mind the better way—is to never, ever put a mushroom in your mouth if you're not 100 percent sure of its identity.

But there will always be some who have to push the envelope of safety. And therein lies the reason that a tiny number of mushroom eaters do get sick or die. Foragers have a saying: "There are old mushroom hunters. There are bold mushroom hunters. But there are no old *and* bold mushroom hunters."

> There are old mushroom hunters. There are bold mushroom hunters. But there are no old *and* bold mushroom hunters.

And in contrast to the many North Americans who are afraid of mushrooms, millions of foragers all over the world eat wild mushrooms throughout their lives without a problem. What's more, billions of people all over the planet eat foraged, wild mushrooms that they've bought in the market or at a restaurant, also without a problem. So you might wonder, "What's going on with these people who get sick or die from eating wild mushrooms?"

There appear to be two categories of these people, and it's pretty easy for you to avoid being in either of them:

- A mishandler of edible fungi
- A careless identifier of poisonous fungi

THREE WAYS TO AVOID GETTING SICK FROM *EDIBLE* MUSHROOMS

(Yes, this is a thing.)

DON'T BE A SLOPPY FOOD HANDLER

A study by the American Association of Poison Control Centers showed that 400 out of 457 adult patients with wild-mushroom poisoning had eaten *edible* mushrooms. So what's going on here? Turns out the mushrooms were mishandled before they were eaten. In many cases, they were stored in a hot car for too long or left on the counter overnight, so bacteria grew on them. You wouldn't do that with store-bought mushrooms or other food, so why do it with foraged food? Always, *always* practice basic, safe food handling. That means store mushrooms in a paper bag, keep them in the fridge, and always cook them before serving.

DON'T GET A RAW DEAL

In some of the cases of correctly identified but incorrectly handled mushrooms described above, the foragers ate the mushrooms raw. So the bacteria colony that these careless foragers grew on their finds in their overheated car wasn't killed off in a glistening pan of hot, melted butter. In Europe, there are several species of mushrooms that are traditionally and safely eaten raw—when handled correctly. But for you, as a novice, a very good rule would be to never, ever eat mushrooms raw—whether from gathering or grocery shopping.

Here's why eating them raw is a problem. Fresh-picked mushrooms—wild or cultivated—are transpiring moisture. In a plastic bag, that moisture will promote the growth of bacteria. If your store-bought mushrooms have flat, brown spots where they touch the plastic—that's bacteria growing on them. That's why it's important to put even store-bought mushrooms in a paper bag in the fridge and to always cook them. Even if mushrooms never see the inside of a plastic bag, there can still be random bacteria growing on anything found in the wild. I mean, you cook all your roadkill before eating it, right?

There are other reasons to never eat mushrooms raw. Popular mushrooms like Chanterelles and Morels contain toxins that break down when exposed to heat. And unless they're cooked, mushrooms are about as nutritious as wood. The fibers need to break down a bit for all the nutrients to be accessible. Allergens can also be a problem. If you don't have a food allergy, you probably know people who do. It's only a small percentage of diners who are allergic to tree nuts or shellfish. Likewise only a small percentage of foragers will be allergic to any given species of mushroom. But for some people, cooking the mushroom for even 5 to 10 minutes destroys the allergens. For others, no amount of cooking will destroy them. Hence the next section.

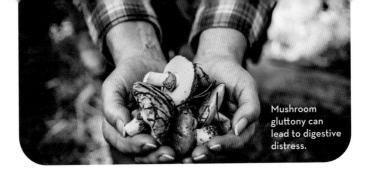

Mushroom gluttony can lead to digestive distress.

DON'T LET A CRITICAL MASS MAKE A MESS

Wild mushrooms are best enjoyed in moderation. Some people will get sick from a correctly identified and correctly handled edible mushroom if they eat too much of it. It's as if the wild mushrooms like to enforce a strict policy against gluttony by humans. Well, of course there's no such policy (that we know of). But it sure is a good idea to act as if the mushrooms on your plate will impose one.

The first time you try a given species of mushroom, limit yourself to a small sample: perhaps 2 or 3 tablespoons, or about enough for an omelet. Within an hour your belly will tell you if you have an allergy to that species. And your uncooked or leftover mushrooms will happily wait for you in the fridge. In the unlikely event you do have some gastrointestinal distress, at least you won't have over-loaded your system. If you feel fine, continue to eat them, but not to excess. A small number of people who've eaten a given edible species many times before can have gastrointestinal distress when eating them in great quantities or if they're undercooked. Note the above-mentioned antigluttony policy.

So, even after you've established that you've handled and cooked your mushrooms properly (just as you would with any food in your kitchen) and that you don't have an allergy, don't make the mistake of thinking you can shovel an obscene amount of deeee-licious mushrooms down your throat. Show some restraint, for crying out loud.

Mushroom Poisoning by the Numbers

Let's get some perspective on the dangers of mushrooms in a country of 330 million people, where the most common sources of poisonings (according to the National Capital Poison Center) are pain medications, cosmetics, and cleaning products. Each of these is 20 times more likely to be ingested than poisonous mushrooms (with or without any symptoms).

THE STATS

Historically, mushrooms account for only about 0.5% (1 in 200) of total toxic exposures reported to US poison control centers. And even that number sounds much worse than it is.

That 0.5% represents a total of 83,140 cases of actual or suspected ingestion of mushrooms that were reported to poison control centers in the United States from 2001 to 2012. Of those, no symptoms were reported in 77% of cases, likely meaning that no one had eaten a poisonous mushroom at all. Only minor symptoms were reported in 13% of cases, likely meaning a bit of food poisoning from edible mushrooms incorrectly handled before serving in most cases.

Moderate symptoms were reported in 9% of cases—probably from the kind of mushrooms that can make you sick, but won't kill you (a.k.a. Sickeners). There were major symptoms in 0.6% of cases, probably either from heavy meals of Sickeners or light meals of Killer mushrooms.

Historically, mushrooms only account for about

0.5% (1 in 200)

of total toxic exposures reported to US poison control centers.

Death resulted in 0.05% of cases (fewer than four deaths per year).
These were mostly from fatal mushrooms, but possibly also a few
cases of the very young or very old or people with weakened immune
systems succumbing to Sickeners or food poisoning.

BAD HANDLING AT RESTAURANTS

According to an analysis by the North American Mycological
Association, "Improper food handling or preparation, rather than
misidentification, has been implicated in almost all cases where illness
from wild mushrooms was traced to commercial establishments
such as restaurants." Here are two examples from this study. In 1987,
five restaurant patrons in Vancouver, Canada, were hospitalized due
to botulism from improperly canned Chanterelles. And in 1991, Morels
served raw sent 77 guests at a Vancouver banquet to the hospital.

HOW NOT TO GET SICK OR DIE FROM POISONOUS WILD MUSHROOMS

In my foraging classes, I like to advise attendees to reconfigure their way of thinking about wild mushrooms. I tell them to—in a sense—stop thinking of mushrooms as dangerous. Think about it: they aren't going to jump into your mouth. And they aren't going to bite you like a snake. In that sense, it isn't really the mushroom that's dangerous—it's the careless mushroom hunter that is. Here are some examples of how to avoid being that dangerous mushroom hunter.

HUMANS AREN'T PERFECT: ERR ON THE SIDE OF SAFETY

We humans make mistakes, because we aren't perfect. (Those of you who are perfectionists need to get over yourselves!) Since we can't identify all mushrooms perfectly, the best thing we can do is decide on which side we want to err. Do you want to err on the side of playing it a bit too safe? Or do you want to err on the side of being risky? Even experts confront this question occasionally.

There are a few mushrooms that defy correct identification in the field or even after consulting guidebooks. At some point we may think, "It's *probably* an edible." And yet we choose to err on the side of being a bit too safe. Why? Because no matter how good a poisonous mushroom tastes (if that's what it turns out to be), a bad outcome just isn't worth it. Come on you guys—we're just talking about some food here. In other words, the eating is not worth the repeating. That is, it will taste better going down than it will coming back up.

So be patient. Other mushrooms that you can identify correctly will show up to replace any dicey ones you toss. Trust me.

YOUR DIPLOMA WON'T PROTECT YOU; GOOD JUDGMENT WILL

You might have noticed that the first half of this chapter wasn't about people getting sick from poisonous mushrooms. And perhaps you thought, "Boy, the people getting sick from correctly identified edible mushrooms are a bunch of dummies." Well, yeah, that's a bit of what's going on. But whether one gets sick from edible or poisonous mushrooms, it's because someone is being a bit of a dummy. (Nothing personal!)

From the title of this section you might think that I don't value intelligence or higher education. But that wouldn't be true. I value education so much that I earned my degree on the Jethro Bodine plan—meaning, I invested 8 years in earning my 4-year degree (if you don't know who Jethro Bodine is, just ask an old person).

What the title really means is that the people who've harmed themselves by not following good protocols around edible and poisonous mushrooms were probably intelligent enough. So clearly it isn't your stunning IQ nor your sterling degrees that are going to save you.

What will save you is the ability to exercise good judgment. If you serve your friends wild mushrooms that make them sick or perhaps risk their lives, most likely you can't blame anyone else. If you don't take the time to properly ID the mushrooms you find, you have no one to blame but yourself.

On the other hand, if you do have a reputation for exercising good judgment, there is no reason you shouldn't be able to learn to gather wild edible mushrooms and share them successfully, for the rest of your long and satisfying natural life.

A person with that sort of good judgment would be one who regularly defers gratification, one who is not out to impress other

Anglophones and Mycophobes

Over time, I've spent what amounts to a year of my life traveling in rural areas of Europe: England, Wales, Denmark, France, Italy, Portugal, and Spain. It dawned on me at some point that it was only in England and Wales that I ran across a general fear of wild mushrooms, which they called "toadstools."

That word actually could be an anglicized German term. In German, Tod, pronounced "tote," means "death." And Stuhl means either a "stool" that you sit on or a "stool" that you poop out. Perhaps it refers to the stool you poop out as you're expiring from a deadly mushroom toxin.

Either way, I noticed that the English stood out in their reluctance to even try mushrooms. This echoed my experience with mushroom hunting in America and Canada (except Quebec). Reading up on Australia and New Zealand, I found a similar cultural avoidance of edible fungi. An Anglophonic mycophobia, if you will.

For a long time I couldn't find anything in the literature that explained this strange fungal factoid.

So I came up with my own theory.

In the days of wooden ships, as English identity jelled on their little island, they began to see themselves as superior to the folks on the continent. This attitude clearly picks up speed after Admiral Drake's tiny navy and some really bad weather crush the Spanish Armada. I suspect that the English were so focused on setting themselves apart that a disdain for potentially dangerous mushrooms—which the inferior continentals were too foolish to avoid—became part of their

Let the eater beware.

identity. I mean, come on, the English are so focused on being different from the continent that they drive on the wrong side of the road.

Having inoculated themselves with the avoidance of toadstools as part of their cultural identity, they then, like a virus, spread that attitude around the globe with their tea, their cricket, and their bossy ways.

Years go by and I come across Gary Lincoff's informative book The Complete Mushroom Hunter. There, on page 11, he mentions his awareness that mycophobia is common in other English-speaking countries, as well as in places formerly governed by Britain including India, Pakistan, and numerous countries in Africa.

But there's more. While mushrooms are avidly eaten in northern Spain, in southern Spain they have historically been feared. And this anxiety spread to their descendants in Latin America along with their colonial ambitions (this despite, or perhaps in spite of, the native populations' fondness for mushrooms).

Where did the aversion to mushrooms in southern Spain come from? No one knows for sure, but we do know the following: During the Spanish Inquisition, authorities outlawed so-called magic mushrooms because they saw them as a tool of the devil. It stands to reason that this religious declaration about one type of mushroom could have had the effect of making all mushrooms—some of which are deadly, and some of which are phallic—seem taboo.

The upshot of all this? The people who love eating wild mushrooms are a vast majority on the planet. And a lot of that mycophobia among the minority has to do with inherited cultural attitudes. Not science. And certainly not taste.

people with foolish acts of daring, one who recognizes that the goal in this effort is self-education and that eating delicious wild mushrooms is the by-product or reward for that education. Basically, someone who eats or shares mushrooms only when they are 100 percent certain of the mushroom's identity.

Perhaps the people who ate bad mushrooms just figured something "natural" wouldn't hurt them. That something "delicious" wouldn't hurt them. That something that "smelled so good" wouldn't hurt them. That something that sort of resembled a half-remembered description wouldn't hurt them. That something that sort of resembled an edible mushroom in their home country on another continent wouldn't hurt them. That something that a wild animal had taken a bite out of wouldn't hurt them (why don't they wonder if that wild animal is perhaps puking its guts out behind a tree somewhere, or is toes-up in the underbrush, or, unlike us, is immune to that mushroom's poisons?).

Poor judgment is really what gets foragers in trouble with mushrooms. So if you have a reputation among your friends and family for exercising poor judgment, then I have to be honest and say that you may not be a very good candidate for becoming a successful mushroom hunter. Not saying that you shouldn't try it. Just saying that I don't want to eat at your house. Perhaps you should pass this book along to a more careful individual of your acquaintance. And then eat mushrooms that *they* gather. Win-win!

SAFETY RHYMES FOR BEGINNERS TO REMEMBER

Until you amass enough knowledge to comfortably consider yourself an intermediate-level forager, I advise using these guidelines to keep you away from many (*but not all*) poisonous mushrooms. There are edible mushrooms that have the features mentioned in these warnings, but detailing all the exceptions is beyond the scope of this little book. As you acquire more books and experience, and move your way up to intermediate or expert status, you'll be able to shed these guidelines as you did the training wheels that helped you learn to find your balance while riding a bike.

What about Spore Prints?

Many mushroom field guides *require readers to take a spore print—which involves leaving a mushroom cap, gills down, on a piece of paper for several hours—so that you can verify its ID by its spore color. In the mushroom entries that start on page 64, you'll notice that spore prints are not always included in the ID checklist. That's because my goal is to teach you to clearly identify mushrooms in the field rather than wait to take a spore print at home. For the cases where the spore color is important for distinguishing an edible mushroom from a Sickener or a Killer, I've included that information.*

WHEN IN DOUBT, THROW IT OUT.

I didn't come up with this catchphrase, but it is the basis of being a safe forager. Any doubt is a reason to do without. I recently heard a colleague voice a similar couplet: "Forget it rather than regret it." And a final one for when you're in the field and don't want to forgo a potentially good find: "When in doubt, let the spores fall out." Only a few of the mushrooms in this book require a spore print to differentiate them from look-alikes. But for those fungi that do demand an overnight spore print or for those anxious foragers who just want to double-check, there's no shame in taking mushrooms home and letting the spores fall out to confirm an ID.

THE EATING IS NOT WORTH THE REPEATING.

Lots of mushrooms that are Sickeners smell appetizing and taste great. But they cause what the doctors call gastrointestinal distress—meaning, those mushrooms will be fighting their way out of your system in one or both directions. I've met people whose enthusiasm led them to mistakenly eat Sickeners. They said the meal was delicious. But no one thought those mushrooms tasted so good as to make them go back for more.

DOES IT HAVE A TUTU?
Eating it's a no-no.

Often the stalk of a soilborne mushroom has a ring around it that resembles a flimsy skirt or tutu. That ring is what's left of the veil that covered the gills when the mushroom first erupted from the soil. There are, of course, some edible fungi that have veils that leave tutus—the only one in this book is the Honey Mushroom—but some of them can be challenging to sort out. Several very

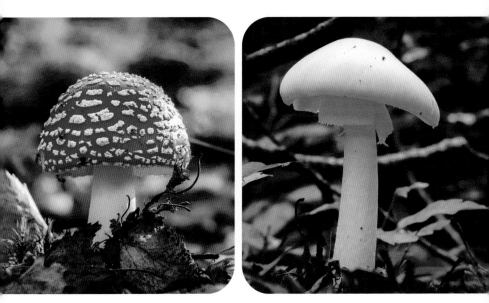

Warts on the cap? A tutu on the stalk? Could be a poisonous Amanita. These two definitely are.

poisonous mushrooms have tutus, such as *Amanita* and *Cortinaria* species, and several fairy ring mushrooms. So, if it has a tutu and you're not 100 percent sure of it, don't eat it.

STALKED, SOILBORNE MUSHROOM CAPS THAT ARE RED OR WHITE?
Just toss it out of sight.

Of course, this means you may be tossing a few edibles at first. But some—not all—of the most poisonous mushrooms fit into this category. None of the soilborne, stalked edibles in this book have red or white caps.

COOL IT OR STOOL IT.

The majority of mushroom eaters who do get sick actually suffer from poor handling of edible mushrooms. That means food poisoning, as you'd get from raw meat left on the counter overnight or restaurant food that's been mishandled. Once you harvest edible mushrooms, treat them like meat rather than a vegetable. You don't need to carry a cooler with you in the woods, but it's not a bad idea to have one in the car if you won't be going straight home. And if you make room in the cooler for your mushrooms by extracting some cold drinks, all the better.

DOES THE SMELL MAKE YOUR HEAD SNAP BACK?
Then don't put it in your sack.

Because one's sense of smell is often more subjective than many foragers are willing to acknowledge (and some people, like longtime smokers, may have completely lost their sense of smell), I don't advocate that novices use their sense of smell to determine a mushroom's secret identity. The same edible mushroom might be variously described as smelling like frozen orange juice or lilacs.

So I recommend taking the descriptions of a mushroom's aroma with a big pinch of fragrant Himalayan salt. Yes, mushrooms may have wonderful or horrible smells, but using these smells for the purposes of identification opens the door to subjective and wishful decision making. And that's where one may find a bit of gastrointestinal distress.

One exception to this is if you find an edible mushroom and your head snaps back when you sniff it—as if you'd sniffed some neglected leftovers in your fridge. That is useful information. It means it's too far gone to be edible. There's no guarantee that you'll

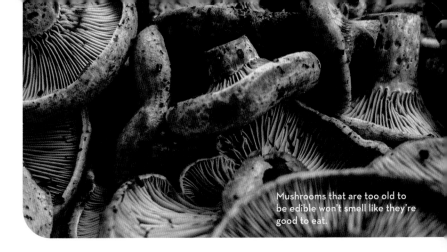

Mushrooms that are too old to be edible won't smell like they're good to eat.

find edibles at their peak of freshness. One thing about the sense of smell that is consistent among foragers, is that once bacteria have had their way, their rank odor will alert you to the danger. Why is this particular scent so reliable? Because all of our ancestors who could *not* discern foods that had gone bad, ate of the fruit of rotten knowledge and died out. Wretchedly. Or perhaps retchingly. And evolution took care of the rest, leaving us lucky ones with the gene for this reliable snap-back safety feature.

NOTE: THESE FEW GUIDELINES DO NOT COVER ALL THE POISONOUS MUSHROOMS OUT THERE.

Not every Sickener or Killer lends itself to an easy rhyme. There are dangerous mushrooms that don't fit these guidelines. But these rhymes allow a novice to skip over a lot of mushrooms that would not reward your investigation with a meal. Conversely, as you acquire more identification skills, you'll find that a few that fit these rhymes are, in fact, edible. However, following the guidelines laid out in these rhymes saves you some time to focus on those edibles that are relatively easy to ID. Consider them as training wheels to help you get started safely.

"Even Experts Can't Tell Them Apart."

Oh really?

Mushroom hunters who are truly careful, exercise good judgment about handling edibles, and toss anything uncertain don't die or suffer gastrointestinal distress.

But sadly, some people will put mushrooms in their mouths that they haven't 100 percent confirmed as edible. There are plenty of legends about "experts" who mistakenly fed poisonous mushrooms to their family. Traditionally in these stories, in the end, all the family members get sick and die. Only the "expert" recovers from the experience, to live on in guilt and infamy. Sounds like a Greek myth.

One example is the story about how the "mushroom expert" and author of the novel The Horse Whisperer served poisonous mushrooms at a dinner he prepared for his wife and her parents. All four almost died; three of them went on dialysis; two of them had to have kidney transplants. In an interview, his wife said he thought the deadly Web Caps (members of the Cortinaria genus) they ate were edible King Boletes. And that her husband's mistake really put some stress on their relationship.

But it gets worse. After eating the Web Caps and feeling ill the next day, they then looked at a mushroom guidebook in their possession and saw their mistake. But the visual differences are painfully clear: The deadly mushroom had gills and a veil on the underside of the cap. King Boletes have pores—the underside of the cap looks like a sponge—and no veil.

I'm sure that author is a nice guy and an outdoorsman as many articles describe him to be. But to mistake fungi with gills for those with pores is not a mistake that an expert mushroom hunter would make. Especially when there's a guidebook sitting around available for confirmation. Sadly, reporters are inclined to describe such a person as an "expert" to heighten the drama of the story (and to boost the number of clicks!).

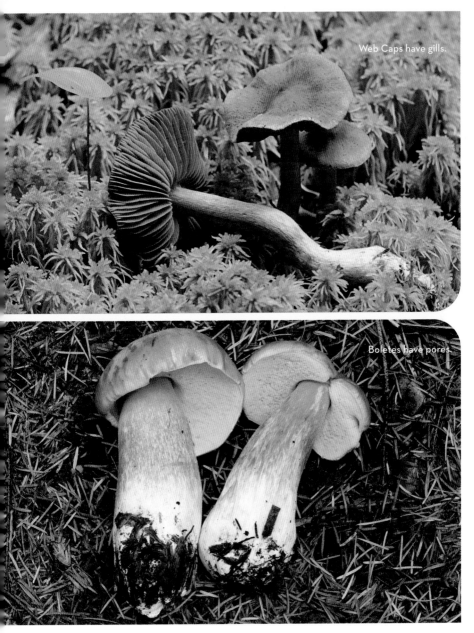

Web Caps have gills.

Boletes have pores.

ELIMINATE THE POISONOUS AND FOCUS ON EDIBLES

The rhyming guidelines in the previous section will be especially helpful if you want to focus your efforts on likely edibles rather than try to ID each of the hundreds, if not thousands, of inedible mushrooms popping up in your region. Use them to eliminate poor candidates, and then use the checklists in this book to nail down the best of the edible fungi. If your find doesn't meet all items on the checklist—toss it. After all this tossing of unlikely candidates, you will still find plenty of delicious, edible mushrooms. And no one will have to get sick.

Using this sort of opt-out list will also spare you from suffering from what I call the 30-30-30 rule. This happens on a mushroom foray when the leader stops to ID every single mushroom a group comes across. It means that you look at your watch and see that in the first 30 minutes of your 2-hour foray, you've only gone 30 feet into the woods and have looked up about 30 inedible or poisonous mushrooms: a fair number of them Little Brown Mushrooms (LBMs; see page 204).

A better practice is to keep moving, gather mushrooms, and then at the end of the foray, lay out a dark fabric in the parking lot for foragers to spread out their finds. The leader can then step back and let the most enthusiastic members scour their field guides and keys to reveal hidden identities.

My practice in the woods when confronted with one of the thousands of mushroom species that aren't edible and would take a long time to ID using a key is to pretend to toss it over my shoulder and say, "Don't know, don't care." Then I pass it back to the finder, ask them to hold on to it, for us to look up at the end of the foray.

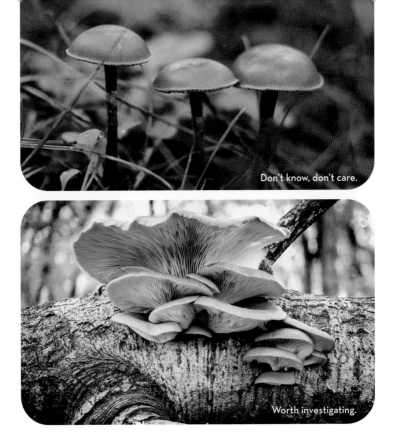

Don't know, don't care.

Worth investigating.

I know the edible, poisonous, and medicinal mushrooms of my area, and unless an unfamiliar mushroom is strikingly beautiful or amazingly weird, I aim to make the most of people's limited time and get us into a big patch of desirable mushrooms as soon as practical. When you're on a tour of a favorite museum, you don't want to lose time examining doorknobs, water fountains, and exit signs.

Life is short. Your foray time is limited. Be focused. Stay safe. Exercise good judgment.

Can You Really Tell a Mushroom by Its Smell?

Our senses are subjective: *They don't give everyone the same information. Red/green colorblindness afflicts 300 million people on the planet. Another 15 million are blue/yellow colorblind. Some people are considered supertasters. And many people who aren't supertasters have told me that mushrooms taste like dirt to them. Smells are certainly subjective and hard to pin down.*

EVERYONE SMELLS DIFFERENTLY

Think about this. Foragers often describe Chanterelles' aroma as evoking apricots. I've smelled apricots. I've smelled Chanterelles. Sorry, but to me they're not nearly the same. Many foragers, when no one's around, have told me they feel the same way.

Since aroma is often unnecessary for an ID, I've kept my mouth shut about it. I used to think that my unrefined palate was the problem. When drinking wine with friends, they notice notes of berries, oak, or the flop sweat of the vintner. But all I'm picking up are hints of grape.

SWEET SCENT OR BURNT RUBBER?

Then I came across Long Litt Woon's powerful memoir The Way Through the Woods: On Mushrooms and Mourning. *Her experience with Chanterelles paralleled mine: no apricots. But experts seemed unanimous that this was the only appropriate descriptor for their aroma.*

Here's her first realization that something was amiss with the idea of fragrance as an ID characteristic: "Some mushroomers describe

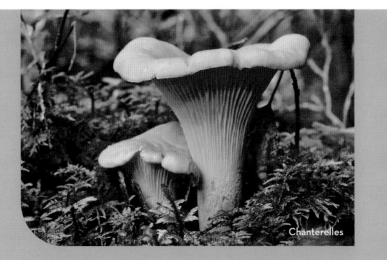

Chanterelles

the Blewit's odor as sweetish and simple. I don't like this mushroom.
I think it smells of burnt rubber. My first teacher described the Blewit's
odor as 'cod liver oil in Wellingtons.'" She describes a years-long
study on mushroom smell she read about in the journal of the Danish
Mycological Society. Among other findings, the study showed that
"an individual's sense of smell also varies depending on their age, on
whether they are taking medications, and for women, on whether
they are pregnant."

Leading a foray of novices to a patch of St. George's Mushroom
(not covered in this book), Long Litt Woon asks them what it smells
like. Their answers: "varnish"; "fresh paint"; "creosote"; "petrol";
"rancid oil"; "walnut"; "mothballs." Their mushroom book described
the smell of St. George's as "wet flour." 'Nuff said.

That's why I don't list aroma as a cue to the secret identity of any
mushrooms. It seems tailor-made to lead an overenthusiastic novice to
declare something safe to eat when it's not. It's time to say that listing
aroma as an ID characteristic should be discontinued.

A WORD ABOUT SUSTAINABILITY

Many people are properly worried about the conservation of endangered species. I am. In my gardens I use native species and pollinator plants to support endangered bees and butterflies. When I was a younger man, I worked one summer keeping the nests of endangered loggerhead sea turtles from being destroyed by raccoons and rising tides. We all have parts to play in conserving wildlife.

Because there are so many threats to endangered species, some people worry that harvesting too many mushrooms may endanger them, too. But that's not something that could realistically happen. Why? Because harvesting every edible mushroom in a plot does no more harm to the fungus itself than harvesting every single apple does to an orchard. The part of the fungus that we like to eat is just a temporary feature that quickly expels billions of spores to seed the next generation before it's eaten by wildlife and/or turns to mush. The body of the fungus—the mycelium—is still living, growing, and multiplying.

The one common exception occurs when foragers harvest mushrooms before they've had a chance to expel their spores. Puffballs are the best example. They are only edible before the spores have developed. So make a point of leaving some Puffballs unpicked (and unkicked!) so they can spawn the next generation and you can live without guilt. Ditto for Lion's Mane. You may find one that has not yet grown any whiskers. The spores come out of the ends of the whiskers, so a bald Lion's Mane is too young to send spores into the world. Come back to harvest it in a few days or a week depending on temperatures. A less common exception is when foragers harvest mushrooms at their button stage or their egg stage. Most mushrooms with caps don't drop spores from their gills or pores until the cap is fully horizontal. With some, you may see a change in the color of the

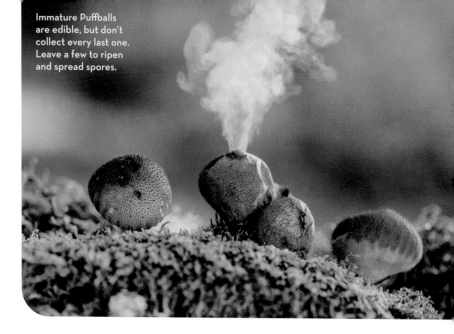

Immature Puffballs are edible, but don't collect every last one. Leave a few to ripen and spread spores.

gills or pore layer that indicates spores have gone airborne. Or you may see the spore color on the caps of lower mushrooms. In those cases you can be confident that billions of spores have already flown on the wind. In any case it won't hurt you to leave some number of the oldest or youngest ones unharvested.

STUDIES SHOW . . .

Thirty-year-long studies in Oregon, Germany, and Switzerland confirm that the production of mushrooms does not decline due to harvesting. The only behavior that seems to inhibit mushroom growth is dense trampling of the ground. In other words, leave the marching band at home when you're foraging. The forest ground can compact enough to inhibit mushroom growth due to lack of oxygen in the soil. But the infrequent and inconsistent foot traffic

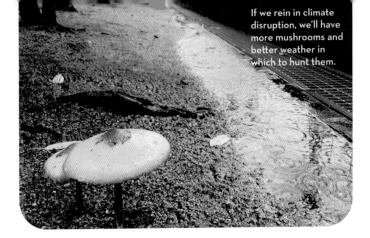

If we rein in climate disruption, we'll have more mushrooms and better weather in which to hunt them.

of mushroom hunters and other walkers is more than balanced out by the work of earthworms and other soil critters that create tunnels and bring oxygen into the soil where fungi can access it.

And because there are thousands of species of mushrooms that wildlife can eat and only a few dozen that humans can eat, we aren't depriving other animals of an important food source. Many insects, reptiles, and mammals have stomachs that denature toxins that would stop us cold.

ANOTHER STUDY

Finland had a modest culture of foraging before World War II. In the 1960s the government hired 22 professional foragers to train 1,600 advisors with the goal of diversifying the food supply and developing new sources of income. These advisors then trained 50,000 pickers to safely identify mushrooms and wild plants. The Finnish Forest Research Institute estimates that now half of the population forages regularly without harming the forests. Many of these foragers have become professionals who sell their mushrooms locally and as far away as Italy.

THE REAL PROBLEM

To the extent that any species of mushroom is in decline, it will come from two sources that have nothing to do with mushroom hunters. The first is development of wild land into neighborhoods, industrial parks, and business districts. As anyone who has gathered mushrooms from their own yards or from park trees knows, mushrooms will find their way; but there are usually fewer species and lower numbers of mushrooms, edible or otherwise, in developed areas.

The other problem is climate disruption. Some people call this global warming or climate change. But both of those terms give some people the false impression that it's no big deal. And to a degree, that's understandable. Word choices matter. Mark Twain pointed out to writers the severe difference between "lightning bug" and "lightning." In terms of the climate, we're dealing with lightning, not lightning bugs.

The reality of climate disruption is that whatever climate you grew up with is gone. And for plants, animals, and fungi in the wild, their territories will shift. I live in the piedmont of central North Carolina. We used to be a good apple-growing region. But the gradual warming trend has made apples a less commercially viable crop here. As temperature patterns and rainfall patterns change, we will be seeing fewer of some mushroom species and more of others, with no guarantee that every good edible we lose will be replaced by something of equal value on our dining room tables.

So if you're concerned about conserving fungi, then inhibiting mushroom hunting would be the wrong way to go. Instead, fight for solutions that leave the open land favored by mushrooms intact. And fight climate disruption every way you can.

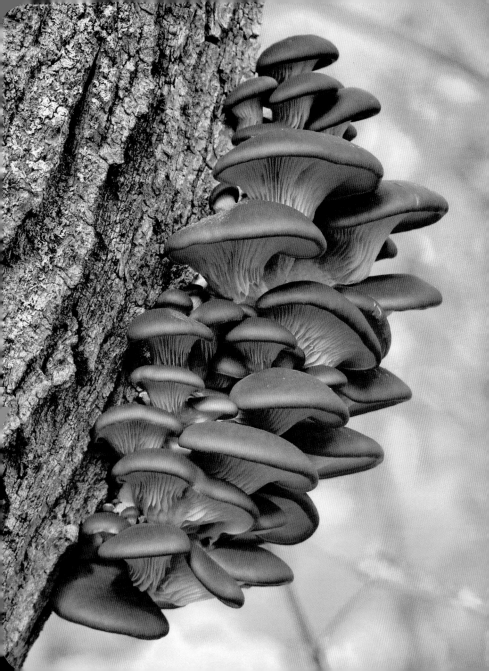

CHAPTER 3

MONEY DOESN'T GROW ON TREES,

but Gourmet Mushrooms Do

Treeborne fungi can be easier to find
than those growing from the ground.
They may be at eye level or higher.
Or near the base of trees or on fallen branches.
They sometimes have bright colors, and
many species are active after tree leaves
have fallen, making them more visible.

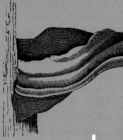

mushrooms without gills
that grow on trees

One way to make the mushrooms in this book easier to find is to separate those that have gills from those that do not. Generally speaking, treeborne mushrooms without gills are safer to start with.

WOOD EAR: Listen Up!

Auricularia auricula

Meaning of the Latin name: ear-shaped, ear

Also known as: Brown Ear Fungus, Tree-Ear, Jelly Fungus

Comparable species: *A. americana* (found in America), *A. angiospermarum* (grows on deciduous trees), *A. fuscosuccinea* (dark amber), *A. polytricha* (many hairs)

As a kid in the woods, you probably first noticed these sturdy yet squishy creatures growing on dead branches. They are common on hardwood in the northern hemisphere. Large ones might be the size of your palm but more often the size of your thumb. They certainly evoke the look of a small human ear just waiting to be nibbled on. And

holding them, they feel almost like those little packets of jelly at a diner.

But perhaps, if you have ever eaten at an authentic Asian restaurant, you have blinked in surprise at finding them floating in your soup. (Lawrence Millman, in his book *Fungipedia: A Brief Compendium of Mushroom Lore,* says that the similar *A. polytricha*—the one smiling up at you from your soup—may be the first cultivated mushroom, grown in China as long ago as 600 BCE.) And they were indeed worth some enthusiastic nibbling then: What they lack in flavor, they make up in a resilient texture.

Having been bitten by the mushroom-foraging bug, you recognize that this wild friend from childhood—now one of your first dinner dates with exotic mushrooms—could be had, free for the taking by anyone careful enough to get the ID right. A couple of species are similar looking, nonpoisonous, and edible, if not as appealing. But let's not get ahead of ourselves.

FEASTING

These taste better than store-bought mushrooms. Slice or serve whole in soup. Braise or poach and slice to serve in salads. There are several reports of it being risky to sauté in an uncovered pan: the moisture inside can come to a boil, exploding the mushroom and making it airborne. No joke. But could be a fun experiment if performed outdoors.

Leon Shernoff, publisher of *Mushroom: The Journal of Wild Mushrooming*, says it can be "ground and mixed with flour to make drop biscuits that puff up tremendously when fried." He adds, however, "Sadly, I do not know the correct proportions to make them puffy, but not explodey."

PRESERVING

Run surplus mushrooms through a dehydrator overnight and store in a glass jar in a dark cabinet. Can be found dehydrated, but still edible, in the wild during dry spells.

FARMING

Can be grown indoors on grain or outdoors on sawdust or logs.

LOOK-ALIKES

Look-alikes are edible—jellylike mushroom look-alikes such as *Tremella foliacea* and *T. mesenterica* (called Witch's Butter) grow on dead branches, similar in most ways to Wood Ear, but all are lacking the tiny hairs on one side and also have one or more of these characteristics: (1) they look like a blob of brains rather than an ear; (2) they look like a snug cluster of leaves; (3) they are brittle enough to break when folded in half; (4) the entire mushroom (or just the underside) is a different color—white, yellow, tan, dark brown; (5) they are sometimes translucent.

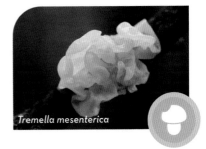

Tremella mesenterica

KNOW BEFORE YOU EAT

WHAT, WHERE & WHEN

- Saprobe on branches of dead or dying trees that still have their bark on.

- White spore print.

- Grows throughout United States and Canada.

- Found in fall, winter, and spring. Also, summer in cooler regions.

FIELD ID CHECKLIST (ALL MUST BE CORRECT)

- Some describe it as root beer colored. Reddish brown to medium brown. Sometimes a hint of violet. Opaque. Blackish when dried out.

- Grows singly or in overlapping clusters.

- Up to the size of your palm, rarely larger, but mostly smaller.

- No stem.

- Surface has smooth but irregular ridges that resemble a human ear.

- Hairless surface on concave side, velvety on the convex side. *Edible look-alikes all lack these velvety hairs.*

- Feels gelatinous. Easily folds in half when moist. Brittle when dry. Similar-looking cup fungi are brittle and will crack.

- The color, texture, and tiny hairs of this mushroom remind me more of a bat's ear than a human ear.

NOTES: *Wood Ear has anticoagulant effects, so don't eat it if you're on blood thinning medications. This list can also be used to ID the comparable species listed on page 65.*

DEVIL'S URN:
Love Me Tender

Urnula craterium

Meaning of the Latin name: little urn, cup or mouth of a volcano

Also known as: Crater's Cup

You're most likely to find Devil's Urn on fallen branches.

The first mushroom hunters

I learned from disdained Devil's Urn as leathery but edible. So I ignored it for years—until I found a young and fresh-looking cluster. These dozen fungi were covered inside and out by a surface of black velvet, smooth enough to serve as the background to a painting of Elvis in a white jumpsuit. Or perhaps a clown crying over a failed Morel foray. They surprised me by being tender to the touch—not stiff, as I'd experienced before. A knife sliced them easily from their oak baton. We'd had plentiful rains the preceding month and the stick looked fresh and intact, although dead. Perhaps

the combination of (1) fresh wood to decompose, (2) plentiful rain to fill out its cells, and (3) being found not long after fruiting presented us lucky foragers with tender tasty Devil's Urn for the first time.

FEASTING

Sliced thin and sautéed in butter, these reveal a tender, meaty texture and rich mushroom flavor.

FARMING

Its reputation for being unpalatable keeps it from being of interest as a cultivated product, but since it grows on wood, it's likely it could be farmed. Cultivation would make it easy enough

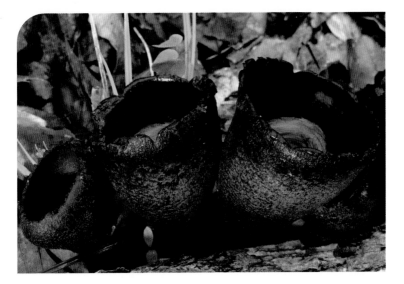

Eat it young and tender, not old and leathery.

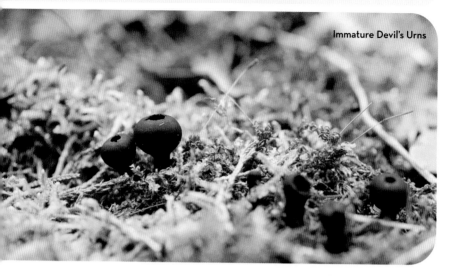

Immature Devil's Urns

to grow in ideal conditions and harvest at peak tenderness. Perhaps it's an unexploited culinary opportunity. Its rich black color, urnlike shape, and meaty texture could inspire chefs and flummox some experienced foragers.

LOOK-ALIKES

There are no look-alikes, but apparently some people want to confuse Devil's Urn with Black Trumpets (*Craterellus cornucopioides*; see page 157). But Trumpets fruit in summer and fall, Urns in spring. And Trumpets are very narrow like a telescope and Urns are wide . . . like an urn. Even if you get it wrong, they are both edible.

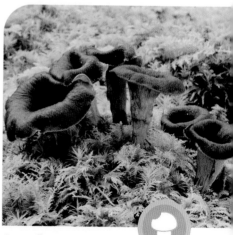

Craterellus cornucopioides

WHAT, WHERE & WHEN

- Saprobe that decomposes dead wood.

- Usually found on sticks on the ground in deciduous forests.

- White spore print.

- Found east of the Rockies, but a very similar member of the genus—
  U. hiemalis—is reported in Alberta, Canada, and in Alaska.

- Early spring, before and during Morel season.

FIELD ID CHECKLIST (ALL MUST BE CORRECT)

- Growing in groups on wood on the ground, but the wood may be
  buried under leaves or soil.

- Shaped like a cup with a wide bottom and sometimes a narrow base;
  tender when young, stiff when older.

- Depending on the amount of rainfall and degree of decomposition
  of the wood, cup may be just small enough to enclose the tip of your
  pinky finger or big enough to swallow your thumb.

- Interior of cup will be velvety black.

- Exterior of cup will also be velvety black when young, but will age
  to an unappetizing, crusty, leathery pink, brown, or black.

- Upper edge may be scalloped or ragged.

NOTE: *This one is edible for a brief period when it's young and tender enough,
after plentiful rains. But if it feels stiff to your fingers or looks beaten up by the weather,
it's likely going to be too tough to be enjoyable. I suspect that difference in age
and conditions explains the conflicting views about Devil's Urn's palatability among
mushroom hunters.*

PHEASANT BACK:
Animal, Vegetable, or Mystical?

Polyporus squamosus

Meaning of the Latin name: many pores, covered in scales

Also known as: Dryad's Saddle, Cucumber Mushroom

During Morel season you'll be looking down at the ground. A lot. But all that glitters is not poking up through fallen leaves. Pheasant Back mushrooms grow on trees and often fruit at the same time as Morels. Take breaks while Morel hunting and refresh yourself with a neck roll, while scanning the trees for these ripening mushrooms. You might also be lucky enough to spot a late-sprouting Lion's Mane or a froth of Oyster Mushrooms spilling from a live or dead tree.

Pheasant Backs grow big and bright enough that they can be glimpsed from a car window on a country road. That's how I found a reliable patch when visiting my wife's family in rural Maine in June. Knowing where it will be, I often catch it while it's young, tender, and nearly the size of a dinner plate. Or five. It flushes from the same spot on a standing dead tree that has shed its bark and identity. When I slice them off the tree I get a whiff of watermelon rind. Some people smell cucumber. But by now you know that mushroom fragrances are just an ephemeral pleasure of life, not an ID characteristic (see page 56).

The peeling scales on top look like a pheasant feathers—if the bird's head were stuck in the tree. Dryads are another name for mythological tree nymphs. And the funnel-like curve of this polypore does evoke the smooth shape of a well-crafted horse's saddle: one sized for a nymph on a midnight ride.

FEASTING

These are tastier than store-bought mushrooms. Young Pheasant Backs are tender enough to eat except for the area around the stalk, which can still be used for broth. On older, larger specimens, the flesh gets tougher, especially the closer it is to the wood. Size doesn't always indicate age. A big,

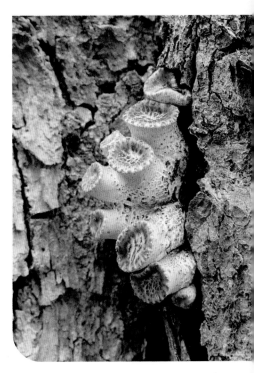

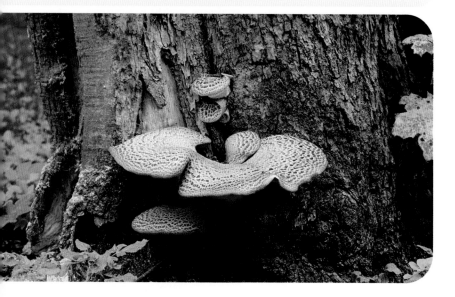

fast-growing specimen may be young and tender, while a small, slow-growing one may be old and tough. On young specimens, the angular pores will be about the size of a pinpoint—just barely visible—and they will scrape off the cap easily. On older specimens, the angular pores are much wider (the size of a pinhead) and the pore layer doesn't come off easily.

Some recipes advise peeling off the top layer. Some advise scraping off the pore layer. I've had good luck so far leaving both in place and slicing off the tree as much of the cap as feels tender.

PRESERVING

Sauté in fat and then freeze. Don't thaw. Throw straight into a hot skillet to finish cooking.

FARMING

It's a decomposer (saprobe) and spawn has started to become available online for cultivation.

LOOK-ALIKES

None.

KNOW BEFORE YOU EAT

WHAT, WHERE & WHEN

- Parasite on living trees. Or a decomposer on dead trunks, logs, and stumps. Mostly on elm and tulip poplar, but also other deciduous trees.

- White spore print.

- Plentiful east of the Rockies. Less common on the West Coast.

- Spring and early summer. Sometimes found in fall.

FIELD ID CHECKLIST (ALL MUST BE CORRECT)

- Fan-shaped or kidney-shaped polypore on a very short stubby stalk.

- Cap may be smaller than your palm to larger than your outspread hand.

- Cap is one or two fingers thick.

- One or more caps, sometimes overlapping.

- Top of cap covered by concentric rows of thin, peeling dark brown scales.

- Pale tan to pale yellow upper surface.

- Underside is whitish and covered by visible pores that are angular, not circular.

- Tender white flesh when young. Less tender with age.

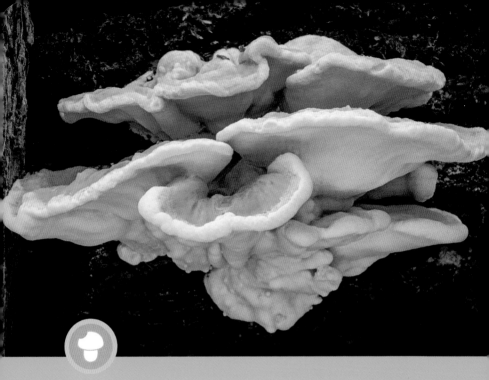

CHICKEN OF THE WOODS: It Really Does Taste like Chicken

Laetiporus sulphureus

Meaning of the Latin name: bright pores, yellow color of sulfur

Also known as: Chicken Mushroom, Sulfur Shelf, Spring Chicken (when found early in the season), Chicken of the Hood (when found inside city limits)

Comparable species: *L. cincinnatus* (named for Cincinnati)

You might find a Chicken of the Woods as a single shelf of a few pounds or a cluster of shelves weighing as much as 50 pounds, or anything in between. It might be growing high enough to require a ladder or on the ground at the base of the tree. The color varies but is always striking: panic orange, cadmium yellow, or, less commonly, a pastel salmon color.

If you're lucky, you'll find it at its most tender: still growing and slightly dewy. In most cases you can grab a shelf with both hands and gently wiggle it until it releases from the tree. Otherwise cut the tender portions away from the tree (*L. sulphureus*) or the ground (*L. cincinnatus*) with a knife.

I'd heard many times that the mushroom called Chicken of the Woods tasted like chicken. I wanted to know the truth.

I got my answer at the Asheville Mushroom Club's big annual weekend of forays and feasts some years ago. Someone handed me a small plate with bite-size pieces of Chicken of the Woods in a luscious tomato-cream sauce. At the first bite I knew the truth. If someone had told me with a straight face that this was a plate of chicken, I would have swallowed that story as fast as I could fork up another bite. It had the very same taste and texture.

FEASTING

This is a gourmet mushroom. Rinse it under the faucet while hand-shredding it into bite-size pieces (it tears like cooked breast meat). Serve well cooked in a soup, stew, or sauce. Or let it cool and prepare as you would chicken salad. Tear it into bigger pieces if you want to grill it, slathered in marinade. Or bread it and fry it. And then invite your friends over for dinner.

PRESERVING

The texture becomes chewy when dried and rehydrated, so sauté first and then freeze. Then don't thaw it out, just cook it.

FARMING

Can be cultivated by inoculating stumps or large logs outdoors.

LOOK-ALIKES

There are no poisonous look-alikes on deciduous trees, but similar-looking species growing on evergreen trees (conifers and eucalyptus) may be inedible, cause gastrointestinal distress, and/or have resinous flavors. *Piptoporellus* species, which grows on live oaks in coastal North and South Carolina, may have a surface resemblance, but its interior flesh is orange and corky.

WHAT, WHERE & WHEN

- A polypore and saprobe that consumes dead wood on live or dead trees, standing or fallen.

- White spore print, but the mushroom may be too old to eat by the time you see spores.

- Most common on oaks but also on chestnuts, beeches, and other hardwoods.

- Both species are often described as only common east of the Rockies. But California-based mushroom expert David Arora describes *L. sulphureus* as "widely distributed and common . . . in our area."

- Mid-spring to late fall. Will likely return each year.

FIELD ID CHECKLIST (ALL MUST BE CORRECT)

- Growing on or right under deciduous trees, especially oaks.

- Semicircular shelflike shape, but also resembles ripply pizza crust.

- As wide or wider than your outspread hand.

- May be stacked on the tree like pancakes.

- *L. sulphureus* grows up trees, has a striking panic orange upper side and a cadmium yellow underside. Upper edge may also be yellow.

- *L. cincinnatus* grows at the base of trees and has a striking pastel salmon upper side and a pale cream underside.

- Undersides of both species covered in tiny pores.

NOTES: *Be sure to confirm your tree species. Any species of Laetiporus growing on an evergreen conifer or eucalyptus tree can make you sick. And, for a small portion of the population, even Laetiporus species on deciduous trees can cause some queasiness. So make your first portion a small one. Some may benefit from cooking this mushroom for a longer period.*

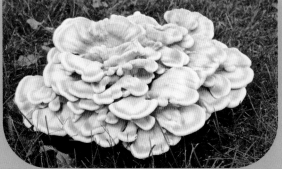

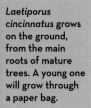

Laetiporus cincinnatus **grows on the ground, from the main roots of mature trees. A young one will grow through a paper bag.**

Chicken Marries Paper Bag

At the base of a tree *near a playground full of middle school–aged boys I discovered a Chicken of the Woods too young to pick. I know what I would have done to a strange object on the ground when I was that age: kick it.*

To spare myself that loss and the mushroom that indignity, I brought a paper grocery bag from my truck, ripped it into a flat shape, and anchored it over the mushroom with a few stones. Presto: My find was disguised as trash too commonplace to be worth kicking.

Returning a couple of days later, I saw that my subterfuge had been a success and the mushroom had grown larger. So large it had grown through the paper bag at several points. I carefully looked for holes in the bag, but there were none. The cells of the mushroom had identified the paper bag as being a wood product: They could penetrate it at a microscopic level. (I love science!) The mushroom and the bag were married wherever they touched. When I lifted the bag in order to harvest, the outer portions of fungus stayed attached to the paper. The paper easily separated from the inner portion of the mushroom without damaging either one. I've started carrying paper bags in my truck on purpose now. I want to see if this works with other species.

BEEFSTEAK MUSHROOM:
Say "Ahhh!"

Fistulina hepatica

Meaning of the Latin name: little pipes, liverlike

Also known as: Beef Tongue, Ox Tongue Fungus

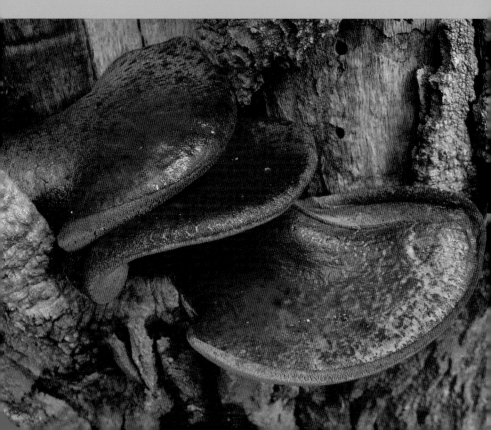

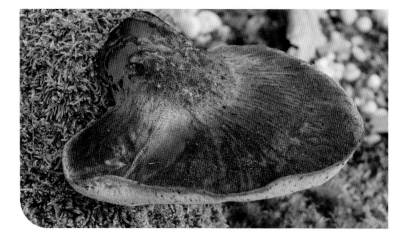

One of the first rules I learned as a novice forager was always cook mushrooms before eating them. But by definition, all rules have exceptions. Beefsteak Mushroom—one of my favorites—is exceptional in many ways. It looks like meat, sometimes bleeds red juices, and can be eaten raw like steak carpaccio.

The reason both wild and cultivated mushrooms should be cooked are several: (1) a raw mushroom is as nutritious as wood, (2) a tiny percentage of people may be allergic to a given mushroom and cooking reduces or eliminates allergens, and (3) whether from the store or the woods, mushrooms can be coated with bacteria, especially if they've been stored in plastic or left in a hot car.

Beefsteaks are an exception to that rule because they are saturated with citric acid, which is what gives them a wonderful lemony scent and flavor. And, as you may know from reading the ingredients lists on packages of food, citric acid is added as a preservative because it deters bacteria. Some plants and fungi use citric acid as a defense mechanism. So a young, tender Beefsteak Mushroom will be free of bacteria. And bugs.

They are also called Ox Tongue Fungus and in fact they do look like an ox hidden inside a tree is sticking its tongue out at you. They are considered a shelf mushroom for their horizontal shape and don't have any poisonous look-alikes. They also have some other virtues. Woodworkers value the "brown rot" that Beefsteaks cause, which makes the wood even more beautiful and valuable. Some foragers lay this fungi upside down on

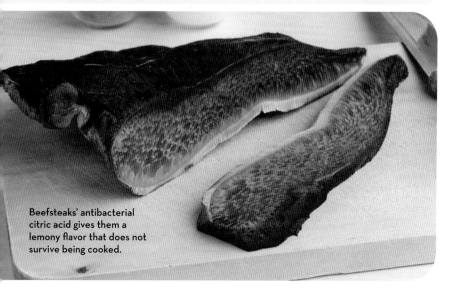

Beefsteaks' antibacterial citric acid gives them a lemony flavor that does not survive being cooked.

tough cuts of meat for a few hours in the fridge; the citric acid leaks out and tenderizes the meat.

Following the rules, I did cook a couple of slices of the first one I found and regretted it. The lemony flavor and bright colors disappeared. Those slices became olive drab with a very mild mushroom flavor. Not appetizing. After confirming with a colleague the advisability of eating Beefsteaks raw, I used the remaining dozen slices to top off a mixed salad. Fabulous flavor and texture. I'd even say it was exceptional.

FEASTING

Slice thinly and serve in a salad or as a substitute for beef in a carpaccio dish.

PRESERVING

Soak it in water with salt and pepper, then run through a dehydrator for faux beef jerky.

FARMING

Can be cultivated on fresh logs or stumps.

LOOK-ALIKES

None.

WHAT, WHERE & WHEN

- Saprobe that decomposes dead wood on live or dead trees.

- Polypore, pores on bottom of bracket.

- Salmon pink to pinkish brown spore print.

- Solitary or several together.

- Late summer to late fall east of the Rockies. Fall and winter west of the Rockies.

FIELD ID CHECKLIST (ALL MUST BE CORRECT)

- Can be as wide as your outspread hand and about as thick as one or two fingers.

- The smooth top will be a delightful pinkish red meat color.

- The smooth underside will be the palest pink/almost white color, disturbed only by the pinkish stain left where your fingers touched it.

- Look closely at the underside and you'll see and feel pores that are separate, individual tubes like tiny straws.

- Flesh is tender.

- When you slice it, you will be shocked by what appears to be streaky bacon. No other mushroom resembles that. Sometimes "bleeds" reddish juice.

REISHI: The Mushroom of Immortality

Ganoderma lucidum

Meaning of the Latin name: lustrous skin, shining

Also known as: Lacquered Bracket, Mushroom of Immortality, Varnished Conk

Comparable species: *G. curtissii* (named for Moses Ashley Curtis, a nineteenth-century mycologist), *G. oregonense* (found in Oregon), *G. tsugae* (found on hemlock trees—whose genus name is *Tsuga*)

Seeing a Reishi mushroom for the first time will convince you that there are fairies in the woods. And they spend evenings painting these mushrooms with shiny reddish brown shellac. Using bird feathers as brushes, no doubt. At its peak of color and sheen—often in late summer or fall—Reishi is as mesmerizing as a campfire. But because they are so dense, tough, and dry, you may see older, duller specimens sticking around for up to a year.

Those who value Reishi's ancestral medicinal properties will pay as much as a dinner on the town for a pound of the dried specimens. Asian apothecaries have sold Reishi for millennia. In Traditional Chinese Medicine, Reishi has been used to support the immune system as well as to fight problems like fatigue, allergies, insomnia, and depression, among others.

FEASTING

While young, the outer edge may be cream or pale yellow. Some foragers find these growing edges tender enough to eat, but the real appeal of Reishi is in steeping it in hot water to make a medicinal tea that some rank as highly as ginseng.

Michael Kuo, author of *100 Edible Mushrooms*, uses Reishi as the base for what he calls his Elixir of Spiritual Potency. He says he can't vouch for its medicinal value but says it hasn't hurt him any either.

He cuts fresh Reishi into ¼-inch slices. It's tough, so use caution. He puts these in a jar, to which he may add other medicinal herbs: cedar berries, spicebush berries, rue, tansy, bay, cloves, and mint. He covers the ingredients with cheap rum and lets it sit for at least a day, though it will store at room temperature indefinitely. He also makes a simpler version with just the Reishi, spicebush berries, and a bit of maple sugar for sweetening. He advises that whatever you do, it's still "a bitter concoction best sipped from a small glass like grappa." So let's lift a small glass to your health. And to the varnish fairies.

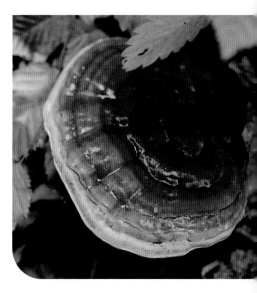

This lacquered mushroom is best in liquor.

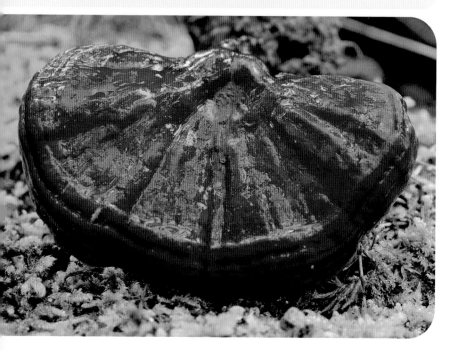

PRESERVING

Dried slices can be stored in jars or kept in alcohol.

FARMING

Tradd Cotter, in his book *Organic Mushroom Farming and Mycoremediation,* considers Reishi "easy to fruit indoors and outdoors anywhere in the world." His book also includes a "mycobrew" recipe for Reishi Red Lager.

LOOK-ALIKES

There are no poisonous look-alikes— no other mushroom looks like it's coated in dark red varnish. Be aware, some mushrooms do look shiny when wet from rain. But even when dry, Reishi is shiny enough to be in a commercial for furniture polish.

WHAT, WHERE & WHEN

- Polypore and decomposer of wood in live or dead broadleaf or evergreen trees.

- May also be found growing from the ground where a tree stump has been ground down or rotted away.

- Brown spore print.

- Single or clusters on same tree or stump.

- Throughout North America.

- Summer and fall. But older specimens hang on throughout the year.

FIELD ID CHECKLIST (ALL MUST BE CORRECT)

- They have a periscope-like stem when young that disappears as they mature into a broad shelflike cap with little or no stem.

- Cap may be as small as a chicken egg or the size of a dinner plate or larger, but most commonly the mature mushroom is the size of your hand and about as thick.

- Upper surface is shiny reddish brown when young with concentric ripples. Outer edge may be creamy white.

- Underside and flesh are white to brownish as it ages.

NOTE: *This list can be used to ID the comparable species listed on page 84.*

ARTIST'S CONK:
Teas, Tattoos, and Tinctures

Ganoderma applanatum

Meaning of the Latin name: shiny skin, flattened

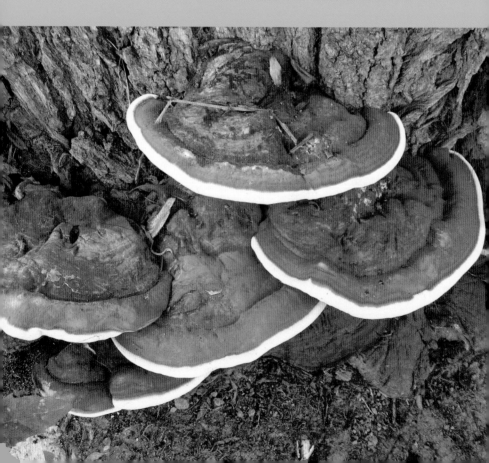

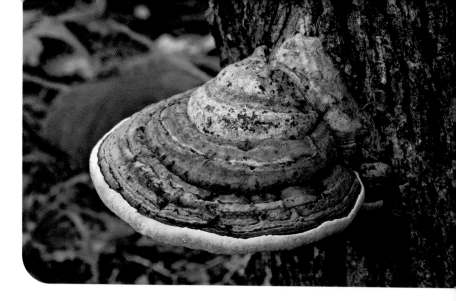

Edible mushrooms are an ephemeral joy: the immediate pleasure of finding and identifying them; the joy of cooking and serving them to friends; the mouthfeel and flavor. And then they're gone except for the memory.

Artist's Conks are different. Their pleasure is a perennial one, though not a culinary one. They are too tough to eat, but it's their toughness that makes them last. And you want an Artist's Conk to last, because its tender underbelly will display a sepia-toned tattoo when you scratch an image onto it with your fingernail or a sharp stick. My sketching skills are modest, but I've had good luck replicating friends' faces from photos.

Remove Artist's Conk from the tree by pushing down on the upper surface (you don't want to mar the tender underside) with both hands. Gently, slowly wiggle it until it loosens and comes off the tree. Continue to protect the underside from contact until you are ready to draw. Make your drawing that day, before it starts to dry out. Untreated, it will last several years before insects find it.

They can be too dry and hard to etch in winter. So come back in spring. They add a lower layer each year, so they get a bit wider with age. Like a tree, you can count the rings on the top surface to estimate how many years it has been growing. Reportedly, new conks regrow from spots where they have been harvested. An Artist's Conk may live for decades, if its tree host lasts that long.

Scratch a sepia-toned tattoo onto its tender underbelly.

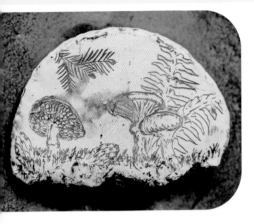

FEASTING

This one isn't considered edible by most people on this continent; even the youngest are too bitter and too woody to eat. But in Asia it's used to flavor soups and drinks. Sometimes it's gathered for use as a medicinal tea or tincture for Traditional Chinese Medicine. It has also been used for dyes, papermaking, felting, and smoking mosquitoes away.

Our primate relatives liked it, too. Primatologist Dian Fossey wrote that for gorillas it was a "delicacy" that they liked to gnaw on—if they could keep it from being stolen by other gorillas.

PRESERVING

To use for medicinal purposes, dry the mushroom and run it through a meat grinder, not a blender. I've read of people preserving their conk as artwork long term but have yet to find detailed information.

FARMING

There are some reports of Artist's Conk being cultivated in the same way other *Ganoderma* species (such as Reishi) are.

LOOK-ALIKES

Red-Belted Polypore (*Fomitopsis pinicola*) looks somewhat similar, except for the distinct red edge on its bracket. Fortunately, it's also considered medicinal.

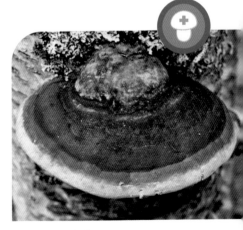

Fomitopsis pinicola

KNOW BEFORE YOU EAT

WHAT, WHERE & WHEN

- Saprobe on living or dead trees, stumps, logs of almost any species, hardwood or conifer.

- Perennial polypore growing from wounds in live trees.

- Bracket shape with pores on the lower surface.

- Brown spore print.

- Alone or stacked in groups.

- Perennial that can be found year-round.

FIELD ID CHECKLIST (ALL MUST BE CORRECT)

- Fan-shaped, semicircular bracket protruding from the trunk like a plate or a shelf.

- Size commonly from dessert plate to large dinner plate. Rarely as wide as your arm is long.

- Thickness ranges from that of a hand to an arm, depending on age.

- Flesh is corky, stiff, and brown.

- Upper surface has shades of dull gray in winter and brown in summer due to spores. Sometimes a lighter-colored margin. Perhaps a dusting of chocolate-colored spores from brackets higher on the tree (the Japanese call it "powder-covered monkey's bench").

- Upper surface covered by wrinkled, concentric ridges that correlate with each new year's growth, similar to tree rings.

- Underside has barely visible pores in a very smooth surface, dull white to pale tan with age. Adds a new layer of pores each year.

- Underside is easily and clearly drawn or written on like a natural, stretched canvas. With a sharp object, or even a fingernail, fine portraits and landscapes can be drawn. These medium-brown markings—stains—contrast with the dull, white pore surface.

EGG NOODLE MUSHROOM:
A Way to Convert Mushroom Haters

Sparassis crispa

Meaning of the Latin name: torn pieces, wavy

Also known as: Cauliflower Mushroom, Ruffles, Wig, Brain Fungus

Comparable species: *S. herbstii* (named for a mycologist), *S. spathulata* (spatula), *S. americana* (found in America), *S. radicata* (has a taproot)

As I've shared wild mushrooms with friends over the years, I've had one unfortunate discovery: the large number of people who find the textures of mushrooms unappealing. The good news is that several wild mushrooms have textures that can convert a mushroom hater into a myco-curious eater. Both Lion's Mane and Hen of the Woods have a meaty density. Oyster Mushroom can be sautéed long enough to make its deep gills crispy. Chicken of the Woods has the mouthfeel of white meat chicken. And Cauliflower Mushroom—despite its name—has the texture and look of yummy egg noodles.

There are several species of Egg Noodle Mushroom in North America. Some people describe their appearance as being like a head of lettuce or a carnation's petals. I think they most closely resemble a big pot of egg noodles prepared by a tribe of small wood sprites—which is exactly what they taste like when cooked. And, given the ambivalence that so many diners have over mushrooms *and* cauliflowers, let's make an executive decision to drop that unhelpful, yet common, cauliflower moniker. I've taken to calling them Egg Noodle Mushrooms, and I think you should, too. With a name like Egg Noodle Mushroom we can change the

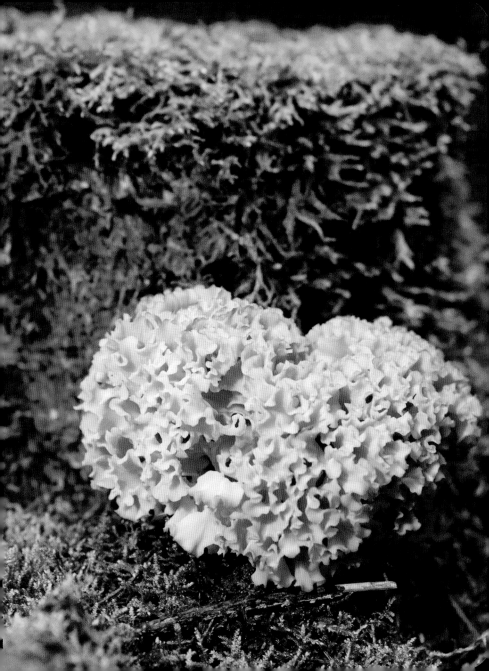

world. Or at least we can persuade a few mushroom haters that fungi can be comfort food, too.

Egg Noodle Mushrooms aren't rare, but neither are they as common in most places as say, Puffballs or Chanterelles. But they don't have to be. One Egg Noodle Mushroom can weigh several pounds and be the size and shape of a small or medium watermelon.

FEASTING

These are gourmet! They can stay in a paper bag in the fridge for as long as 2 to 3 weeks if you want to save them for that dinner party with your fungi-fearing friends. The presentation of a steaming serving bowl full of what

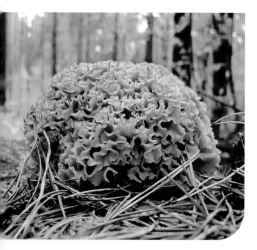

looks like butter-slicked egg noodles can be very disarming. Your guests may briefly forget their unfounded fear that you're trying to poison them. And their childhood memories of a favorite comfort food will wash over them instead.

Best to pick when the "noodles" are whitish. The yellower they get, the tougher they can be. But I've eaten them with a mild yellow tint and the texture was terrific, so that varies.

Break one up by hand as you clean it under the faucet and sauté for 5 to 10 minutes in butter and salt: Taste as you go and cook until al dente. West Coast species may need to cook longer to get a tender texture.

PRESERVING

I've never found more of this mushroom than could be eaten right away, but Antonio Carluccio, in *The Complete Mushroom Book*, says that he has "preserved it in oil, frozen it and dried it, all with excellent results."

FARMING

From inoculation to fruiting time on stumps or buried logs can be 1 to 2 years according to Tradd Cotter in his book *Organic Mushroom Farming and Mycoremediation*. Indoor cultivation is rarely successful.

LOOK-ALIKES

None.

WHAT, WHERE & WHEN

- Saprobe (or sometimes parasite) on wood and roots at the base of dead or dying trees.

- White spore print.

- Singles, rarely groups, at the base of mature hardwood trees or conifers.

- East of the Rockies in summer and fall. West of the Rockies all fall and into winter.

FIELD ID CHECKLIST (ALL MUST BE CORRECT)

- Size and outline of a small or medium watermelon. Rarely, can be much larger, up to 50 pounds.

- Composed entirely of densely branched, flat, ribbonlike lobes that resemble egg noodles attached to a sturdy base.

- White noodlelike lobes when young, that with age become pale yellowish and then perhaps tan.

- Western species may have a deep, hard root in the ground.

NOTE: *This list can be used to ID the comparable species listed on page 92.*

HEN OF THE WOODS: This Hen Nests between Tree Roots

Grifola frondosa

Meaning of the Latin name: intricate like a woven fish basket, leaflike

Also known as: Maitake (Japanese for "the dancing mushroom")

Half the time I see Hen of the Woods, it looks like a clump of fallen leaves piled up against the trunk of a mature oak tree. That's why I rarely worry about people snagging "my" Hens. They sprout from the same trees every fall, but they are well camouflaged. Hens are one of the best, meatiest, wild, edible mushrooms. Sorry to say, they aren't found west of the Rockies. But they're almost enough reason for someone on the Left Coast to move to the Other Left Coast.

The overlapping fronds supposedly resemble overlapping feathers and are responsible for the name. It's no relation at all to the Chicken of the Woods. Totally different mushrooms.

The gourmet, meaty texture makes these very popular with chefs. They're also good for converting people who claim to be "mushroom haters." I break up and roast Hen of the Woods in a way that each frond is like a boneless short rib that can be dunked in a savory dipping sauce. This is a really good mushroom for nostalgic vegetarians who miss the texture of meat.

GATHERING

Before picking one up, check that there isn't a fire ant nest under it—one forager of my acquaintance had to learn that the hard way. Reach underneath with both hands. Rock it back and forth till it comes loose from the soil. Scrape or cut away any debris on the bottom. Store in a paper bag.

FARMING

As a saprobe, it feasts on dead wood, so can be cultivated on oak sawdust and buried oak logs.

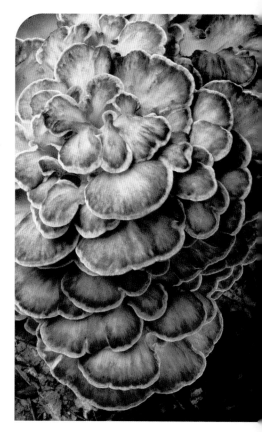

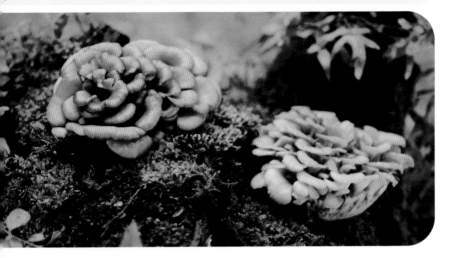

PRESERVING

Cut or tear into small drumstick-size pieces. Spread on a baking sheet—so they don't freeze in a clump—and put in the freezer. After a couple of hours, pop the pieces into a freezer bag. Don't thaw. Simply pop them into a hot skillet and start cooking. This is the rare mushroom that can be frozen raw and the texture won't be ruined.

FEASTING

Rinse and tear apart under the faucet. Dry on a towel. Sauté in butter and seasonings for 10 minutes. Or spread in a casserole, cover with oil, salt, and pepper (as you would for roasting root vegetables), and put in a 400°F (200°C) oven. Stir after 15 to 20 minutes. Roast for another 15 to 20 minutes and serve as a side dish or with a dipping sauce.

LOOK-ALIKES

Hens have several look-alikes that occur at the base of deciduous trees, but all three of them are edible if not nearly as desirable: Black Stainer (*Meripilus sumstinei*), Berkeley's Polypore (*Bondarzewia berkeleyi*), and Umbrella Polypore (*Polyporus umbellatus*). The first one obviously stains black when you damage it. The first two also look more like wiggly spirals of pizza slices than overlapping gray/brown crackers like a Hen. The last one has flat fronds that are lighter colored and much smaller than the Hen's; only an inch or so across.

WHAT, WHERE & WHEN

- A polypore and saprobe that decomposes the dead wood inside a living or dead, large, deciduous tree.

- Grows between the root flares at the base of the trunk or stump, sometimes inside a rotten stump; mostly found on oaks.

- White spore print on older specimens.

- East of the Rocky Mountains.

- End of summer into early winter.

FIELD ID CHECKLIST (ALL MUST BE CORRECT)

- A solid white base with white shoots and tiny pores.

- Shoots grow like broccoli shoots, but are topped by a flat frond smaller than your palm.

- Upper surfaces of fronds are on the color spectrum between dusky gray and light to dark brown.

- Fronds overlap like feathers.

- Entire mushroom the size of a cantaloupe to a very large watermelon.

NOTE: *Hen of the Woods contains tyramine, so people taking MAO-inhibitor medications (a type of antidepressant) should avoid this mushroom.*

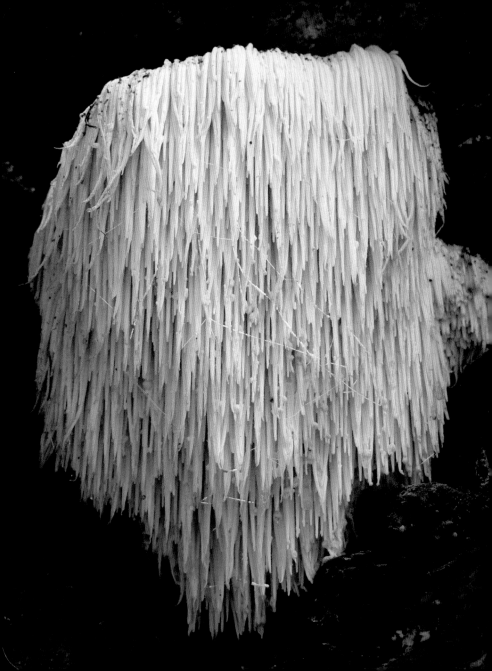

LION'S MANE:
Or Shall We Call It "Santa's Beard"?

Hericium erinaceus

Meaning of the Latin name: hedgehog, hedgehog

Also known as: Old Man's Beard, Santa's Beard, Satyr's Beard, Bear's Head, Deer's Tail, Pom-Pom, Hedgehog (a name now more commonly used for the soilborne *Hydnum repandum*)

Comparable species: *H. coralloides* (like coral), *H. americanum* (from America), *H. abietis* (grows on fir trees)

On my way to visit a friend in the country, out of the corner of my eye I saw a 6-pound Lion's Mane about 20 feet off the ground and 100 feet from the road. After you've seen your first *Hericium*, you'll have these side-eye experiences, too.

Climbing up the wide, straight oak trunk was out of the question. I rode on to my friend's house for help. He had only a 4-foot stepladder. Scouring his garage, I also commandeered a pitchfork and a couple of plastic tubs full of Christmas decorations.

Back under the Lion's Mane, I stacked the two tubs. Then I positioned the stepladder on top of them, leaning it against the tree. With pitchfork in hand I slowly worked my way

up. I did have to come down a couple of times to adjust the tubs or the ladder. I wanted to be safe after all.

With the tubs and ladder stabilized, I inched my way up again. Standing on the top step, I tried to reach the Lion's Mane with the pitchfork, which only reached far enough once I held the very ball end of the handle in my right hand. A lifetime of carpentry work gave me just enough strength in my fingers and forearm to slowly stab the Lion's Mane from the bottom and work the tines farther up. The curve of the tines gave me just enough leverage to pry the mushroom away from the tree. It popped off, fell off the pitchfork, bounced off my shoulder, and fell to the ground. About a quarter of it remained on the tree, but I didn't want to be greedy.

I returned my leaning tower of misfit tools to my friend along with a chunk of my foraged find for his dinner. And resolved to keep a ladder in my truck during Lion's Mane season.

FEASTING

This is gourmet! Kent and Vera McKnight, authors of *A Field Guide to Mushrooms: North America,* shear off the inch-long whiskers, simmer them for a few minutes, and serve them like pasta with butter and dill.

However prepared, the texture of Lion's Mane is less like a rubbery, store-bought button mushroom and more like a piece of blue crab claw meat or a succulent piece of chicken. Its natural

form of monosodium glutamate (MSG) amplifies the other flavors in the dish.

Best to squeeze out excess moisture (see Field ID Checklist) and then dry-sauté hand-shredded portions. That, or braise in liquid. Shredding the flesh by hand gives it the look of crabmeat. The technique many foragers (including myself) prefer is to hand-shred it and use it as a replacement for crab in your favorite crab cake recipe. Form it into patties, fry it in butter, and dip in remoulade sauce.

PRESERVING

Cooking and then freezing maintains the texture. When ready to cook, don't thaw—simply toss frozen bits into the skillet.

FARMING

Grows easily indoors on bags of wood chips or sawdust. On live trees they can only fruit from openings in the bark. On trees with high-fruiting, tough-to-reach Lion's Mane on your own land, it may be worthwhile to drill a few holes through the bark at chest height to see if they'll fruit at a more accessible level.

LOOK-ALIKES

No poisonous look-alikes. But the inedible, pale, hard *Climacodon septentrionalis*—which also grows on trees but has spines showing only on the underside—can give novices false hope.

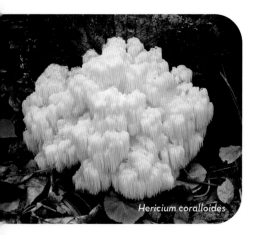
Hericium coralloides

WHAT, WHERE & WHEN

- Saprobe that rots dead wood on live or dead trees, standing or fallen. Sometimes a parasite that attacks live wood.

- White spore print.

- Often high and alone on mature oaks, beeches, maples, and sycamores (*H. erinaceus, H. coralloides, H. americanum*); or on conifers (*H. abietis*). Rarely near ground level unless growing from a cut log.

- *H. erinaceus* and *H. coralloides* found throughout the United States and Canada. *H. americanum* found east of the Rockies. *H. abietis* found in the Pacific Northwest.

- In warm climates: fall, winter, and spring. In cooler climates: summer and fall.

FIELD ID CHECKLIST (ALL MUST BE CORRECT)

- Depending on species, either rounded like a melon (*H. erinaceus*) or branched like coral or furry icicles (*H. abietis, H. americanum, H. coralloides*).

- Downward-pointing spines as long or longer than a fingernail cover almost the entire surface regardless of the mushroom's shape. When very young, spines have not yet formed. Don't harvest then as they haven't yet dispersed spores.

- Bright white at a distance and sometimes up close. Some species have a pinkish tinge. With age the spines may develop a buff color, but that does not necessarily mean it has lost its wonderful flavor or texture. But if yellowing on the inside, it may have developed a sour flavor.

- From the size of a fist to as big as a small sheep. More commonly the size of a cantaloupe.

- Tender flesh of *H. erinaceus* can be twisted like a sponge to release excess (and flavorful) water over a bowl. Like a sponge it will return to its original shape.

Finders Keepers
Fungus Eaters

The voluptuous mushroom grew out of a hollow in a vast oak tree. Grew? It billowed out of the hollow like a toasted meringue waterfall. To reach it, I had to mount the top plate of my 8-foot yellow stepladder that for some reason said "Do not stand here." My chest pressed against the tree. I looked up and stood beard to beard with the bottom half of a Lion's Mane mushroom. I'd only ever heard of this mushroom growing to the size of a soccer ball or football. But this creature was the size of a sheepdog.

I was thrilled and anxious. Could I safely yank this huge, high-dollar mushroom off the tree without becoming a fall guy for this fungi?

I can't truly say I found this mushroom. Truth is, it was found for me.

I was attending my first meeting at a local photography club, sitting in the back row while images flashed on a screen: close-ups of flowers and animals at the zoo. Then I saw a close-up of a Lion's Mane mushroom. I leaned forward and salivated like one of Pavlov's dogs.

The guy sitting in front of me said, "This is a nasty fungus growing on a tree in the woods near my house." Then he showed a wide-angle shot of the mushroom on the tree. I couldn't speak. I heard a murmur among the 40 or so photographers: "Ewww, nasty fungus."

Afterward, I told the photographer that the fungus was a gourmet mushroom: "If you tell me where it is, I'll get it and share it with you." With disgust he said, "I'll tell you where it is, but you can have the whole damn thing."

The 3-inch blade of my pocketknife wasn't nearly long enough. Anticipating this problem, I had borrowed my wife's good bread knife. She wouldn't mind.

I started cutting the bottom fifth off as a start. The mushroom was dense but yielding: like cutting through a pillar of filet mignon or a cheesecake.

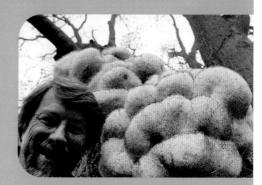

I had thought five paper grocery bags would be plenty, but it was barely enough. Each bag was so full it looked like a fat man wearing a skinny man's T-shirt.

It dawned on me that perhaps I had snagged a mushroom worthy of the Guinness World Records book. But I had no scales to weigh it. And no witnesses. The lonely life of the forager. (Turns out the biggest Lion's Mane ever recorded was twice this size, anyway.)

Scratching my own beard, I pondered my next steps.

As a farmer 35 years ago, I used to barge into restaurant kitchens to sell my organic tomatoes. I felt confident about pitching to a chef. But I'd never sold mushrooms before and had only been foraging for a year.

In 2 hours, I sold 29 pounds of Lion's Mane to five chefs in downtown Durham. I made enough money to buy a month's worth of groceries. I did keep 4 pounds to eat and share with friends.

I was proud of my fluky foraging success. But I wondered if it meant I'd peaked early as a mushroom forager. Would it all be downhill from here on out?

TINDER CONK:
Tinder for a Fire,
If Not a Romance

Fomes fomentarius

Meaning of the Latin name: tinder, kindling

Also known as: Tinder Polypore, Touchwood Conk, Firestarter Mushroom, Horse Hoof Fungus, Iceman Polypore, Amadou, Surgeon's Agaric

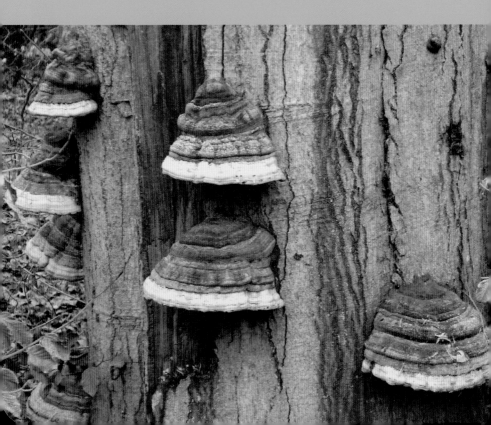

Tinder Conk has been used to start fires, burned as incense, and to stop bleeding.

It looks suspiciously like a horse's hoof, but it's been used for almost everything except making glue. Tinder Conk has been found at Stone Age sites that date as far back as 11,600 BCE. The felty material inside the Tinder Conk has been used to start fires, burned as incense, and to stop bleeding. Sometimes called "German felt," it has been used to make hats and vests. It's also considered a medicinal with antibacterial and anticancer qualities.

Tinder Conks are perennial mushrooms that may live 30 to 50 years. So only harvest them if they are plentiful and you fully intend to make use of them. You will have the best luck tapping them with a mallet to remove them cleanly from the tree.

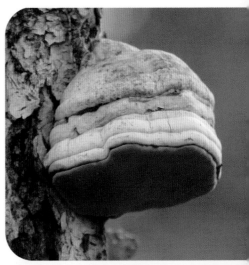

FEASTING
It's not commonly eaten, but it can be used as a medicinal; it has been used as a diuretic and a laxative. But you may appreciate its capacity for stopping bleeding.

PRESERVING
Air-drying will keep it stable indefinitely.

FARMING
According to Tradd Cotter's book *Organic Mushroom Farming and Mycoremediation,* "Harvested conks

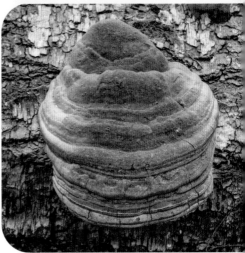

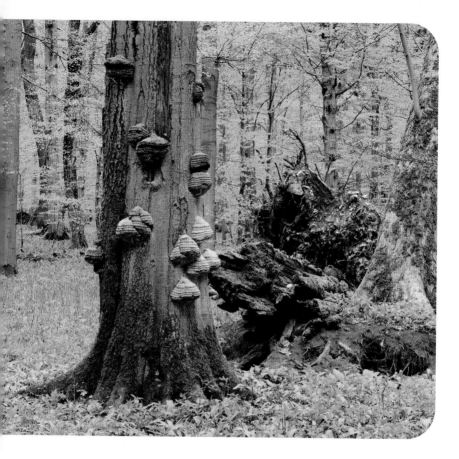

can be submerged upside down in water, weighted down to keep them from floating, with the attachment point sticking up above the water and capped with wet cardboard. Mycelium leaps to the cardboard in one week, giving you viable samples to plant into downed trees and stumps by wafering (inserting small pieces of the cardboard into wounds created with a machete or hatchet)."

LOOK-ALIKES

None.

WHAT, WHERE & WHEN

- A parasite of live trees and a decomposer of dead trees, standing or fallen.

- White spore print, but only drops from spring to fall.

- Found mostly on birch, but also beech, maple, and poplar.

- Can be found throughout Canada and the United States, but more common at higher elevations and cooler regions.

- Perennial that can be found year-round.

FIELD ID CHECKLIST (ALL MUST BE CORRECT)

- Shape resembles a horse's hoof.

- Easily visible horizontal ridges (that tell the conk's age, like so many tree rings).

- Cap hard and woody, often gray, but also gray-brown and sometimes black.

- Underside flat, smooth, cream colored to brown, darker with age.

- Interior hard, fibrous, and cinnamon colored.

- Can range from the size of your fist to longer and wider than your forearm.

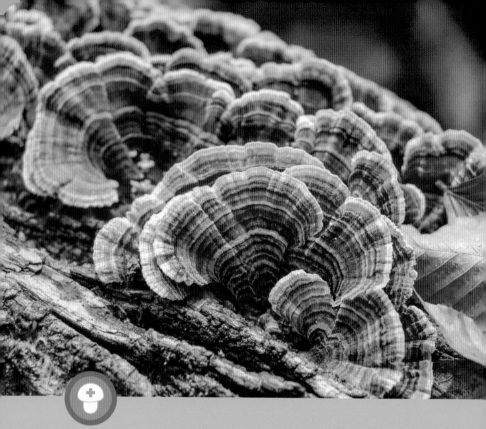

TURKEY TAIL:
Bright Colors, Powerful Tea
Trametes versicolor

Meaning of the Latin name: thin, many colors

Also known as: Many-Colored Polypore. Because of its overlapping growth pattern, in Japan it's called *kawaratake*, which means "roof tile mushroom."

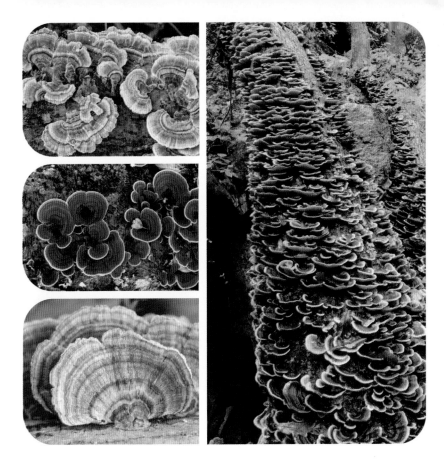

A mushroom hunter in Virginia gave me my first taste of Turkey Tail tea. Her name had been given to me by an acquaintance and forager of wild plants a few counties over. But I don't remember her name; a clear indication that I need to start taking mushroom-based memory enhancers.

We left her cabin and walked around the woods a bit looking for mushrooms. Few were out except Turkey Tails and False Turkey Tails, sometimes on the same log. She showed me how easy it was to sort them out: The underside of False Turkey Tail is smoother, darker, and has no pores.

Like most foragers I've known, she was generous with her time. We went to her kitchen as we swapped stories. She pulled dried Turkey Tails from a jar in her cupboard and tossed a big spoonful in a pot of water on a low boil. She said she varied the amount of time depending on the aroma, how stressed she was feeling, and even how busy she was. Because its earthy flavor is a tad on the bitter side, she offered maple syrup to sweeten my cup of tea, dark as Earl Grey and robust as Turkish coffee.

FEASTING

It's not considered an edible mushroom because of the leathery texture, but in *Organic Mushroom Farming and Mycoremediation*, Tradd Cotter says that "dried brackets can be powdered into flour for adding to breads, soups, pastas, and sauces." Some foragers use it like bay leaves to season a soup and then remove them.

It's most commonly used for medicinal tea or tincture. Some studies indicate that it has antitumor and antioxidant properties, and it reportedly boosts white blood cell counts after chemotherapy. If you're on medication, check with your doctor about possible interactions.

PRESERVING

Dehydrating the mushroom pieces and storing them in a jar in a dark cabinet will keep them indefinitely.

FARMING

Since it's a decomposer, commercial spawn can be purchased on grains, sawdust, and wooden dowels for outdoor cultivation on logs or wood waste.

LOOK-ALIKES

False Turkey Tail (*Stereum ostrea*) has a completely smooth, pale brown undersurface. Hairy Bracket (*Trametes hirsuta*) has a coarse, hairier cap and grayer colors with a brownish edge.

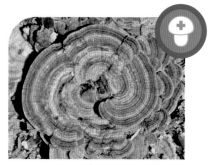

Stereum ostrea

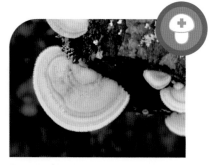

Trametes hirsuta

KNOW BEFORE YOU EAT

WHAT, WHERE & WHEN

- Saprobe that decays sapwood of dead trees.

- Shelflike polypore.

- White spore print.

- In woodland. On stumps, trunks, and fallen branches of dead hardwoods, mostly oak trees. Rarely found on conifers. Said to be the most common species of shelf fungus in the world.

- An annual polypore, but long lasting, so visible in any season.

- Fruits in winter and spring in western states. Summer and fall east of the Rockies.

FIELD ID CHECKLIST (ALL MUST BE CORRECT)

- An individual shelf may be the width of your thumb pad to the width of your palm.

- Overlapping fan-shaped. Sometimes forms rosettes.

- Thickness of heavy cardstock. Leathery.

- Flat or wavy edges with velvety upper surface.

- Lower surface is white with visible pores. This is the most important feature for distinguishing from look-alikes, which don't have pores.

- Concentric stripes of several colors ranging from brown, blue, and green to red. Always a whitish margin.

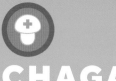

CHAGA:
The New Ginseng?

Inonotus obliquus

Meaning of the Latin name: fibrous ear, slanting sideways (the latter is a reference to the pores of the fertile body, which grow infrequently and appear under the bark of the tree, not on the actual conk)

Also known as: Clinker Polypore, Birch Canker, Birch Conk

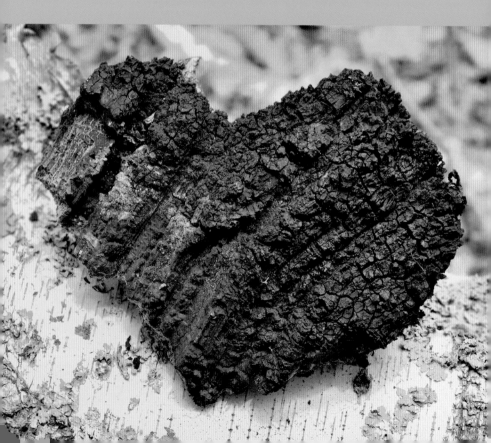

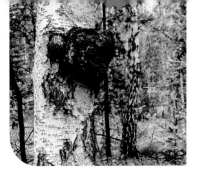

Walking down a woodsy trail one summer in Maine, forager Parker Veitch pointed out birch trees that had been scarred by errant snowmobiles in winter. Soon we found a crusty, black, watermelon-size canker of Chaga fungus growing out of a waist-high scar.

To show me his technique, Parker pulled out a hatchet and broke off only the outer half of the Chaga. He pointed out that collecting all of it was a too-common practice and a good way to kill the tree by leaving a point for infection. By leaving much of the Chaga intact, he knew he could come back in a few years and harvest more.

Chaga looks like a gnarly piece of charcoal sprouting from a tree trunk. Break it open and the inside looks like orange-brown wood. Its size can range from 4 inches to 4 feet across. It has tiny pores rather than gills. It's commonly referred to as a "conk" mushroom like other dense mushrooms that grow on trees, such as Artist's Conk and Tinder Conk.

Chaga prefers to grow on white and yellow birches but may also be found on elm, alder, and beech trees. There is an energetic debate as to whether the Chaga is helpful to the tree or is destroying it. We'll have better answers to these kinds of questions when the food industry has spent as much money studying fungi as they have spent on studying fruits and vegetables.

To preserve the tree, one shouldn't harvest Chaga that's smaller than a grapefruit or while the tree's sap has started running in late spring. You will get the highest levels of medicinal qualities if you harvest it when the tree is dormant in fall, winter, and early spring. But if you find it in summer and know you won't make it back when the tree is dormant, it won't hurt to harvest it then.

Native people of North America and northern Eurasia have used it for millennia as a clothing dye, kindling, and, most often, as a source of medicinal tea that boosts the immune system. A Chinese monk in 100 BCE described Chaga as "the king of herbs" and a "precious gift of nature" (this from the land of ginseng). Aleksandr Solzhenitsyn mentioned Chaga as a cancer remedy in his book *The Cancer Ward*.

FEASTING

The beneficial ingredients only become available after exposure to hot water—as a tea or added to coffee—or to alcohol when making a tincture. It's not bitter the way many medicinal mushrooms are. I've steeped it, strained it, and enjoyed it as a tea without needing sweetener or milk. Boiling it for 2 hours is recommended. But out of sheer laziness I mostly add it to coffee grounds and let the coffeemaker do the work.

In his book *Edible and Medicinal Mushrooms of New England and Eastern Canada*, David Spahr describes successfully using Chaga as a replacement for hops in his homebrew. Chaga can also be made into an alcohol-based tincture.

If taking any medication, check with your doctor for possible interactions. Start with a small dose.

PRESERVING

When I get some Chaga home, I take a hammer and chisel and break the dry, dense fungus down to pieces the size of chicken eggs. I've also put it in a plastic bag and driven my truck over it on the concrete driveway to quickly break it up into egg-size or smaller chunks. Drop two or three pieces at a time into a high-speed food processor and pulverize it to the consistency of coffee grounds. It's best to dedicate a food processor or coffee grinder to this task so you don't irritate your spouse. (Don't ask me how I know this.)

Alternatively, if you missed your workout, you can shred it by hand with a cheese grater. Or run it through a gristmill. Store the powdered Chaga in an airtight container. Bring a 5:1 ratio of water and Chaga to a boil, then let steep for a couple of hours. Filter and serve or store in the fridge.

Some foragers add it to their hot chocolate. I toss a spoonful of ground Chaga per mug on top of the beans in our coffee grinder. It complements the flavor of coffee, adding mild notes of vanilla or nuttiness. And memories of the Maine woods.

FARMING

Not yet propagated.

LOOK-ALIKES

Not really. There are often tumors on trees, but they are covered by bark. On trees in the cherry family, the toxic black-knot fungus (*Apiosporina morbosa*) looks a bit like Chaga, but it is small and grows on twigs. So learn the difference between birches and cherries to be safe: Birches have peeling bark and cherries have horizontal lines of dashes and dots in their bark.

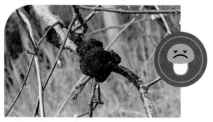

Apiosporina morbosa on a cherry tree

KNOW BEFORE YOU EAT

WHAT, WHERE & WHEN

- Perennial, starts as a parasite and then develops into a saprobe. Found on living or dead trees.

- Erupting from one or more hollows in mature white, yellow, and black birch tree trunks at any height.

- More common on older trees.

- Mostly on birch, less often found on beech, hornbeam, elm, and alder. Those on birch have the most medicinal properties.

- Found east of the Rockies and north of the Carolinas.

- Reportedly, needs to be above a certain elevation, but I've found no data on that. It may be more an issue of needing cooler temperatures and being particular about tree species.

- Can be seen year-round, but is best harvested when temperatures are below 40°F.

FIELD ID CHECKLIST (ALL MUST BE CORRECT)

- Found on birch trees.

- Exterior brittle, crumbly dark brown to black. Resembles charred firewood. Very hard.

- Interior corky, hard, and crumbly yellow to golden brown. Sometimes bits of white. May resemble rotten wood.

- Shape and size irregular and vary from round baseball to flattened watermelon to lumpy goat head.

- Can only be removed with a hand ax or saw.

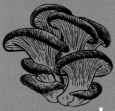

treeborne mushrooms
with gills

As a novice, I heard several times that mushrooms growing on trees won't kill you. Although this isn't true, what *is* true is that edible, gilled mushrooms can be found on trees in any season—even in winter.

OYSTER MUSHROOMS:
Easy to Find, Delicious to Eat
Pleurotus ostreatus

Meaning of the Latin name: ear on its side, oyster

Also known as: Tree Oyster

Oysters make a perfect reward for the novice forager: easy to spot, easy to identify, and they taste great, too. You may be able to find cultivated Oyster Mushrooms at your farmers' market and get a good look at them before foraging for wild ones.

When a friend wanted me to teach him to forage, we walked across the road from his property into some woods. Less than 50 feet in, Oysters greeted us on a big fallen beech tree. We both grabbed double handfuls to bring home. We spent more time preparing and eating them than we spent foraging. You may not always find Oysters so quickly, but they are very common in the woods.

Most edible mushrooms grow on the ground, where they may be small, few in number, obscured by leaves, and hard to find. An Oyster Mushroom, on the other hand, may only be a few inches across, but Oysters often grow in clumps the size of a soccer ball. And they are up off the ground, making them among the easiest mushrooms to find.

FEASTING

This one is gourmet, though unfortunately, Oyster Mushrooms get their name from their appearance, not their taste or texture. The dense, white flesh has a straightforward mushroom flavor, although some people detect a mild licorice scent on the fresh ones. My wife isn't fond of the texture of mushrooms generally, but I found a cooking method that had her asking for seconds of Oyster Mushrooms; see page 221.

PRESERVING

Oysters can be dried and stored in jars, but their reconstituted texture can sometimes be leathery. More reliable results can be had by cooking and then freezing them. Don't thaw. Just throw them into a hot skillet.

FARMING

Perhaps the easiest mushroom for novices to grow. Can be grown on coffee grounds (the heat has sterilized the substrate!) in a bucket in the kitchen.

LOOK-ALIKES

Some *Crepidotus* species, such as *C. applanatus,* look somewhat similar but are smaller, have no stem, appear more often as individuals, and have a brown spore print. Angel Wings (*Pleurocybella porrigens*) are thin and white, but grow on conifers. Neither look-alike should be eaten.

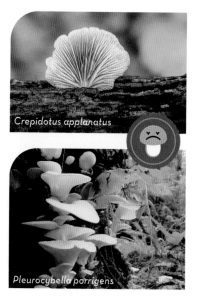

Crepidotus applanatus

Pleurocybella porrigens

WHAT, WHERE & WHEN

- Decomposer on live or dead deciduous trees, standing or fallen.

- Clustered, overlapping rows.

- White to pale lilac spore print.

- Throughout North America.

- Oysters grow year-round, even in snowy winters. In warmer weather they grow fast, get buggy, and pass their "harvest-by date" pretty quickly. So best harvested in cooler weather.

FIELD ID CHECKLIST (ALL MUST BE CORRECT)

- They project out from a deciduous tree trunk or stump.

- Caps the size of your palm to fully outspread hand, sometimes larger.

- Each individual mushroom overlaps two mushrooms below it, like shingles on a roof.

- Gills continue along the stem.

- Gills are white.

- Stubby stem doesn't rise to meet the center of cap as with most gilled mushrooms; it comes off from the side.

- Smooth cap color ranges from bright white to gray to brown, making them stand out from the darker bark of the deciduous trees they grow on.

RINGED HONEY MUSHROOMS:
The Mafiosi of Mushrooms

Armillaria mellea complex

Meaning of the Latin name: ring/bracelet, honey

Also known as: Oak Root Fungus, Shoestring Root Rot, Bootlace Fungus

Comparable species: *Armillaria tabescens*

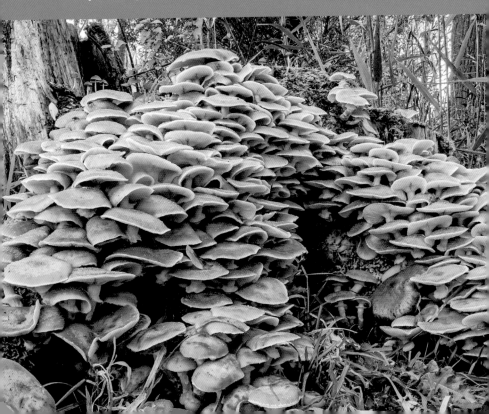

Honeys are called _famigliola_ in Italy, for growing in compact "family" clusters; this can help in their identification. _A. mellea_ is really a complex of about a dozen similar mushrooms with rings on their stalks. They can be popular with novices and others because they are relatively easy to learn and are plentiful when found. They're called Honeys for their color, not their flavor, which compares well to Shiitake.

Another consideration about Honeys is that they can be tree killers. Almost every other edible mushroom is either politely collaborating with tree roots to make its daily bread or is thoughtfully recycling dead wood while leaving living cells undisturbed. They might look sweet, but these Honeys are hungry assassins of trees and shrubs of the forest, garden, and orchard. Knowing that, when I see Honeys near farms and homes, even if I don't intend to eat them, I gather them and toss them in the trash (not the compost) to reduce the spores they can distribute. It is, after all, possible to have too much of a good thing.

FEASTING

Better than store-bought mushrooms (though see Know before You Eat, page 125). Toss the stems, parboil the caps for at least a minute, then slice and sauté the caps for ten minutes to avoid GI distress.

PRESERVING

Parboil, sauté, and freeze. Do not thaw before cooking.

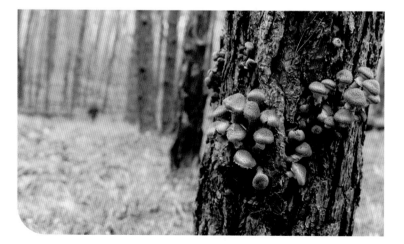

They might look sweet, but these Honeys are hungry assassins of trees and shrubs.

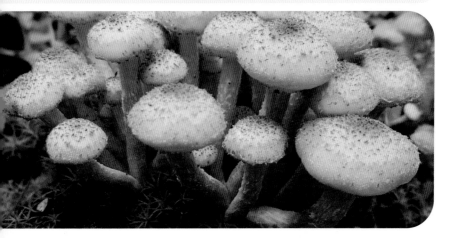

FARMING

They could conceivably be cultivated on live or dead wood, but would you really want to bring an ardent tree assassin onto your property?

LOOK-ALIKES

Ringless Honey Mushroom (*A. tabescens*) has a growth form that resembles Honey Mushroom, but without a veil or tutu on the stalk. It is a saprobe and may be a parasite. It's also edible. Under casual observation, toxic *Galerina*, *Omphalotus*, and *Gymnopilus* species can be mistaken for *Armillaria*, but carefully checking for the spore color, cap color, gill structure, and substrate described in the ID checklist on the opposite page will exclude all three of them.

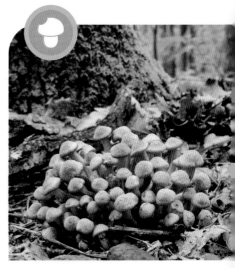

Armillaria tabescens

KNOW BEFORE YOU EAT

WHAT, WHERE & WHEN

- Saprobe of dead wood and parasite of live wood.
- Can be seen growing from live wood, but also seen on the ground drawing from tree roots.
- Fruits in one or more very dense clusters.
- In woods, gardens, orchards.
- Year-round in the West. Summer and fall in the East.

FIELD ID CHECKLIST (ALL MUST BE CORRECT)

- Growing in a dense cluster from a central point.
- Cluster as wide as the size of your fist to as wide as a pizza.
- Growing from wood (aboveground or buried).
- Caps are smaller than your palm, may be sticky, and have tiny hairs on the center.
- Stalks are up to twice as long as your finger.
- Cap color is various honeylike shades of yellow to brown.
- Gills are white, attached to the stalk, and may be covered by a veil that always leaves a tutu around the stalk (unless they are Ringless Honey Mushrooms).
- Young stalks are white, but age to pinkish or brown.
- White spore print.

CAUTION: *For some people, Honeys fall into the "edible-but-forgettable-if-not-downright-regrettable" category. First, the stems are pretty tough; not everyone knows to dispense with them and just eat the caps. Second, it's often recommended to boil the caps before sautéing, to avoid gastrointestinal distress. Third, it's best to eat the very young specimens (a day or two old) while the caps are still cuplike and before they have flattened out. Decay can begin quickly in these species. Fourth, those growing from wood of locust, eucalyptus, hemlock, or buckeye reportedly also cause gastrointestinal distress. Even working around all those considerations, some people still find Honey Mushrooms promote stomach upset. So, cook well all mushrooms that are new to you and eat just a few.*

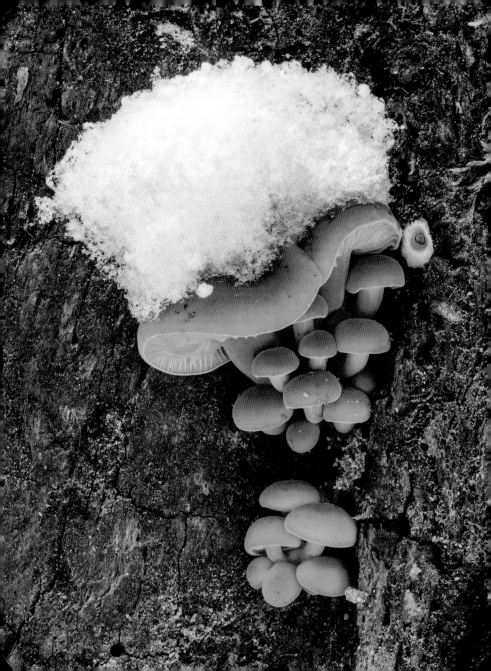

VELVET FOOT:
An LBM Worth Eating

Flammulina velutipes

Meaning of the Latin name: small flame, velvet foot

Also known as: Velvet Shank, Winter Mushroom, Enoki (but the latter—grown for market—is now determined to be a different species of *Flammulina* and looks nothing like the wild one)

Velvet Foot is a great wintertime mushroom, especially in colder regions when there are few edible mushrooms out. It can survive freezing, and even when frozen solid can be gathered and cooked after being thawed out. In warmer regions, foragers may pass them up for more tempting winter mushrooms such as Oysters and Lion's Mane.

Don't let the small size and brown cap bother you. Yes, it fits the definition of a Little Brown Mushroom (LBM; see page 205), but I'm including it here because many rules in mushroom hunting have exceptions. And the nutty flavor of Velvet Foot justifies this one. Plus, I want to give you one more good reason to get out in the woods on a sunny winter day.

The cultivated Enoki mushrooms found in markets have been described as the same species in the past, but now we know that's not the case. Cultivated Enokis resemble long white bean sprouts without a bit of velvetiness.

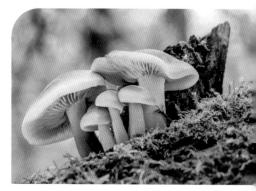

FEASTING

These are better than store-bought mushrooms. Remove tough stalks. Sauté caps quickly—2 minutes—to retain a slight crunchiness for stir-fry dishes.

PRESERVING

Dehydrate and powder in a food processor for long-term storage. Use for flavoring soups, stews, and sauces.

FARMING

What's now recognized as a different species of *Flammulina* and has the common name Enoki can be grown on hardwood sawdust. Grown in low light, it has a very long, slender stalk. The cultivated and wild versions of *Flammulina* do not look at all alike.

LOOK-ALIKES

This mushroom has a velvety stem, but its Killer look-alike, called Funeral Bells, has an iron fist—dispelling the common, yet false, notion that there are no poisonous mushrooms growing on trees. You Latin speakers know it as *Galerina autumnalis* or *G. marginata*. It is a similar size, similar cap color, and somewhat similar growing pattern. Learning to sort out these two works as a marker of a mushroom hunter who's ready to graduate from being a novice to becoming a knowledgeable intermediate forager. So. Pay. Close. Attention. And use the side-by-side checklist on the opposite page to carefully compare their traits before eating any mushroom you *think* is Velvet Foot.

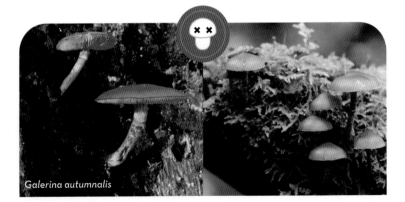

Galerina autumnalis

KNOW BEFORE YOU EAT

WHAT, WHERE & WHEN

- Saprobe that decomposes dead wood.
- Individuals, tufts, and clusters on deciduous trees, sometimes in hollows and under peeling bark.
- Throughout the United States and Canada.
- Fall through spring east and west of the Rockies. Summer in the Rocky Mountains.

FIELD ID CHECKLIST (ALL MUST BE CORRECT)

VELVET FOOT	FUNERAL BELLS
Cap is smaller than your palm, stalk is shorter than your fingers.	Cap is smaller than your palm, stalk is shorter than your fingers.
Velvety hairs (dark brown to black) on lower stalk.	No velvet on stalk.
Gills are whitish to whitish yellow.	Gills are yellow brown to rusty brown.
Flesh is white to yellow.	Flesh is brown.
No ring zone.	Ring zone forms a veil (resembles a tattoo of a tutu).
White spore print.	Rusty brown spore print.

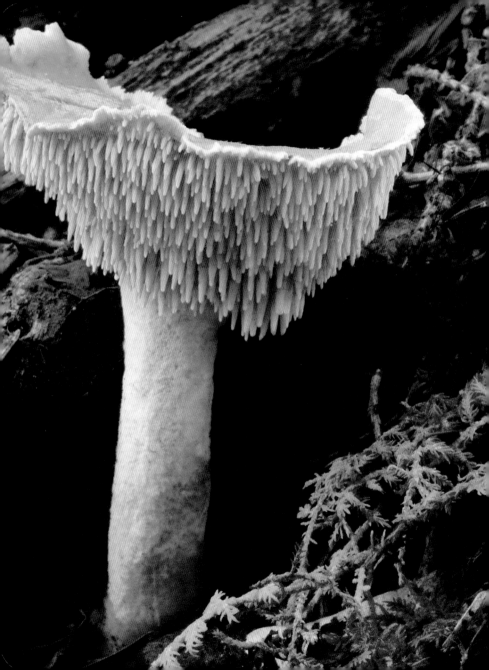

CHAPTER 4

THE FUNGAL FLEET
at Your Feet

In the mind of a novice, the classic mushroom grows from the ground. Some do so because they are decomposing organic matter from dead plants. Some do so because they are collaborating with tree roots. Except in the case of Morels, neither characteristic helps with identification—knowing them just provides a little scientific satisfaction while thinking about mushrooms. But there is one big difference that helps with identification: Some will have gills and some will not.

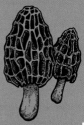

mushrooms without gills
that grow on the ground

Many groundlings without gills have very distinctive ID features, including pores, spines, ridges, honeycombs, or a smooth surface under their caps. Nongilled mushrooms have no Killers among them, but you still need to watch out for the Sickeners.

MORELS:
The Finger Puppet Fungi
Morchella esculenta

Meaning of the Latin name: German for "morel," edible

Also known as: Yellow Morel, Tulip Morel

Comparable species: *M. deliciosa* (delicious) White Morel, *M. elata* (lofty or elated) Black Morel

The mighty Morel is sought after by chefs, professional mushroom hunters, and novice fungus eaters. It's the very best of the few edible mushrooms that fruit in spring. Not only does it have a meatier texture than most store-bought mushrooms, it's relatively easy for novices to learn to safely identify.

Morels somewhat resemble the outline of a cartoon Christmas tree: a fat stalk and a crinkly, conical cap. Cut a Morel in half from top to bottom. Both the stalk and cap have enough of a void that you could almost stick one on every digit like finger puppets. The hollow is also big enough to house a few insects, another reason to slice them open before cooking. As the old folks in the mountains say of Morels, "If it's hollow, you can swallow."

Being a good Morel hunter means being a good tree hunter. The

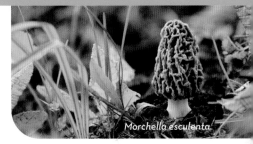

Morchella esculenta

submersed part of a Morel—its inedible, stringy mycelium—grows (in the East) on forest floors in association with tulip poplars, elms, ashes, and old apple trees.

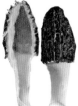

Don't be discouraged if you don't find Morels on your first foray. Most edible soilborne mushrooms announce them-selves across the forest floor like so many brightly colored peri-scopes of yellow, orange, red, or blue. But Morels camouflage themselves quite well. They wear the brownish grays of fallen leaves, with their outline broken up by a shadowy honeycomb of craters in their caps. My technique for finding Morels? Like the commander of a luckless subchaser, I often stop in disappointment and disgust at being empty-handed even though I'm standing among massive tulip poplars. Then I look down at my feet. Half the time, I'm standing in the middle of an under-the-radar fleet of Morels. Then I use my pocketknife to cut them off at soil level (no sense getting dirt in all those craters) and debate the various ways to cook them on the way home.

FEASTING

This is a gourmet mushroom. Chefs and farmers' market shoppers will pay more per pound for fresh or dried Morels than for New York strip steak or filet mignon. And if you've ever had them in a stew, perhaps with venison and ramps, you'd understand why. Best sautéed but can also be added raw to cook in soups, stews, sauces, and on pizzas.

PRESERVING

If you have a surplus, put them in a dehydrator overnight at about 110°F (43°C). That will let you save them in a jar in your cupboard. Rehydrate for a few minutes in warm water before adding to a skillet or casserole. Or just toss dried Morels straight into a soup pot.

FARMING

One Asian species of Morels is a decomposer (rather than a mycorrhizal species, like most Morels) and reportedly can be grown on wood chips. Apparently, however, the texture and flavor leave a lot to be desired.

LOOK-ALIKES

There are a few mushrooms that—with some enthusiastic wishful thinking—look enough like a Morel to earn the name "False Morels," including *Gyromitra esculenta*. These look-alikes are all mostly or partly solid inside, not entirely hollow as a true Morel is. And the top looks more like a brain than honeycomb. If you find those, leave them be. In general, they are unappetizing, and some can play havoc with your digestion. Do not eat them.

Similar-looking *Verpa* species, such as *V. bohemica,* also should not be eaten. One identifying feature is that the bottom of its honeycombed cap ends in a skirt rather than adhering to the stalk.

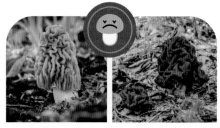

Verpa bohemica   **Gyromitra esculenta**

WHAT, WHERE & WHEN

- Mycorrhizal with tree roots, most often, but not exclusively those of elms, ash, tulip poplars, apple trees, and conifers.

- Individuals scattered or in groups on the forest floor and old apple orchards.

- In the Midwest, Rockies, and Pacific Northwest, Morels respond to the previous year's forest fires with great flushes rising from blackened earth. Unfortunately, eastern Morels haven't learned this trick, making them a bit harder to track down.

- Morels appear in mid-spring, after the last frost, but before the tree leaves come out. They seem to be triggered by a good rain about the time the soil temperature reaches 53°F (12°C).

- Mid-spring in the eastern United States. Mid- to late spring in the Midwest. Early summer in the Rockies. Almost year-round in coastal California.

FIELD ID CHECKLIST (ALL MUST BE CORRECT)

- Dull, gray, brown, or yellow conical cap with irregular honeycombs. May have black edges.

- Bottom edge of cap completely adheres to the stalk.

- Thick, smooth, white stalk roughly the same length as the cap. Hollow and often big enough to insert a finger in many cases.

- Slice in half: Morels are hollow from top to bottom. (False Morels will be mostly solid with just a few voids. Toss them.)

- Morel size may range from the thickness and length of your thumb to the height and width of your flattened hand depending on conditions, age, and species.

NOTE: *This list can also be used to ID the comparable species listed on page 133.*

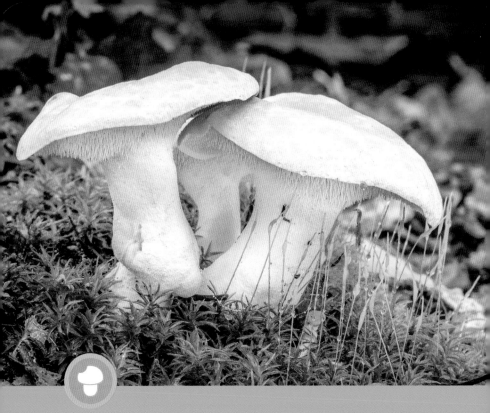

HEDGEHOG:
Hedge Your Bets and Hog Your Share

Hydnum repandum

Meaning of the Latin name: Greek for "truffle" (because of its desirability), cap bent upward

Also known as: Wood Hedgehog, Sweet Tooth, *dentini* (Italy—for its teeth)

Hedgehogs are cousins to Chanterelles and nearly as popular, if not as common. Insects don't seem to like them very much, which is good news, but it's still smart to slice Hedgehogs lengthwise to expel any bugs or dirt that may collect in a central depression of the cap.

They have a mildly meaty texture and a distinct ID characteristic: tiny spines suspended under the cap. The spines are the launch tubes for spores and they have a pleasing texture. Italian foragers call these mushrooms *dentini,* for their "teeth." Those teeth do like to catch dirt, however, so give all mushrooms a good brushing before dropping them in your bag.

Novices will enjoy learning Hedgehogs; They may be the most common toothed mushroom and there are no poisonous look-alikes.

FEASTING

Highly sought after for a texture like Chanterelles (see page 172), gourmet Hedgehogs have a milder flavor.

PRESERVING

Like Chanterelles, they don't rehydrate well. You may want to powder them after drying. Alternatively, sauté and freeze them, or make a conserve, as the forager chef Alan Bergo does (see page 244).

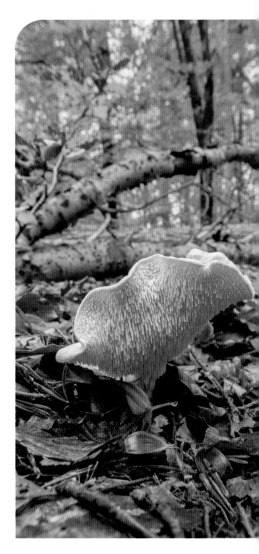

It'll bare its teeth, but it won't bite.

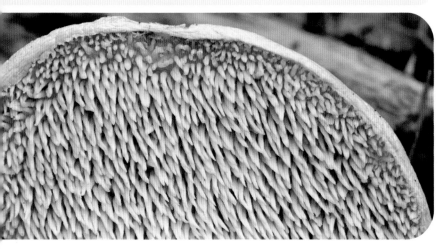

FARMING

As mycorrhizal mushrooms they collaborate with tree roots, so they have not been cultivated.

LOOK-ALIKES

There are two other, similar-sized soilborne mushrooms with teeth under the cap. But where Hedgehogs have brittle flesh, these two are tough and leathery. One is *Sarcodon* species, which is darker and/or has scaly caps and a brown spore color that often darkens the spines. The other is *Hydnellum* species, which is leathery. Neither is poisonous, but neither is palatable either.

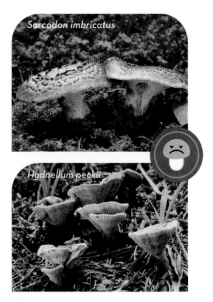

Sarcodon imbricatus

Hydnellum peckii

WHAT, WHERE & WHEN

- Mycorrhizal, generally on broadleaf tree roots in the eastern United States or on conifer tree roots in the Rocky Mountains to the Pacific Coast.

- White spore print.

- Grows on the ground in forests, singly or in small groups. Rarely in large groups or rings.

- Throughout North America.

- Midsummer to early winter in the East, fall in the Rockies, and fall and winter west of the Rockies.

FIELD ID CHECKLIST (ALL MUST BE CORRECT)

- No cup, tutu, veil remnant, scales, or warts on cap or stalk.

- Cap is the size of your palm more or less with a smooth to suedelike top surface. Wavy edges. Pale tan to pale orange color. Cap color can resemble color range of Chanterelles, to which they are related.

- Stalk may be the thickness of your thumb or finger, usually shorter; white inside and out.

- Underside of cap is white and completely covered by teeth, all shorter than a thumbtack. Teeth same or paler color than cap.

- Stains pale orange to brown where touched or damaged.

PUFFBALLS:
Get Your Kicks
Calvatia, Calbovista, and *Lycoperdon* species

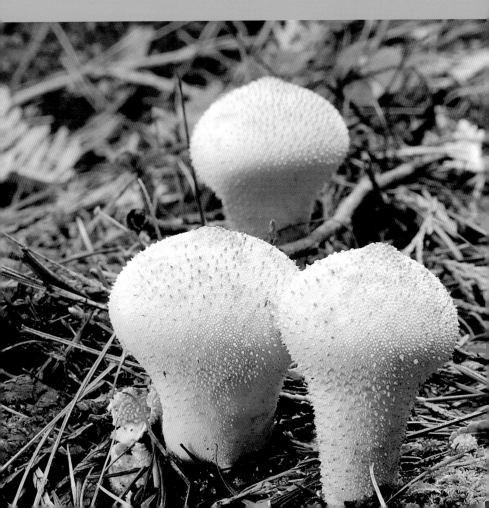

I'll bet you've seen Puffball mushrooms before. As a kid, you probably gave a few of them a swift kick just to see their spores fly. I harbor an unproven theory that Puffballs coevolved with Stone Age children busting these white balloons and unknowingly spreading their spores far and wide.

A Puffball full of dusty spores is certainly fun to play with, but it's too mature to eat. You want to catch them early, before the spores have formed. Cut one in half and if all you see is a soft white substance like tofu, then your timing is right; colors other than white mean it's overripe. If you find the outline of a conventional mushroom inside, it's not a Puffball but possibly a poisonous Amanita. If you see a gelatinous alien creature, it's an immature Stinkhorn. Either way, toss it.

Puffballs are among the easiest edible mushrooms for novices to find and identify. Depending on the species, they range in size and shape from that of a grape to a large watermelon. Most, but not all, have a plain, smooth, white exterior. Rarely, you find one with a bit of gray peach fuzz or short, soft spikes. A few have a geometric, patterned surface, like a fungal braille

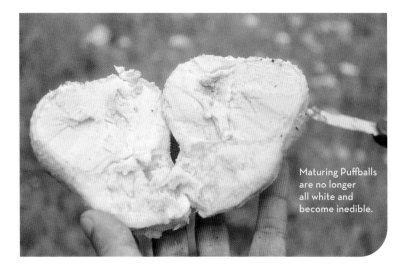

Maturing Puffballs are no longer all white and become inedible.

PUFFBALLS OF ALL SIZES

BIGGER THAN A TENNIS BALL

COMMON NAME	LATIN NAME	MEANING
Giant Puffball	*Calvatia gigantea*	bald, giant
Western Giant Puffball	*Calvatia booniana*	bald, named for W. J. Boone
Sculptured Puffball, Sierran Puffball	*Calvatia sculpta*	bald, sculpted scales
Pedestal Puffball, Purple-Spored Puffball	*Calvatia cyathiformis*	bald, cup-shaped
Sculptured Puffball	*Calbovista subsculpta*	bald-fox's fart, less prominent sculptural scales

SMALLER THAN A TENNIS BALL

COMMON NAME	LATIN NAME	MEANING
Common Puffball, Gem-Studded Puffball	*Lycoperdon perlatum*	wolf's fart, widespread
Peeling Puffball	*Lycoperdon marginatum*	wolf's fart, margin

message. Most of them are linked to their underground mycelium by a dimple at their base, though Pedestal Puffballs or Purple-Spored Puffballs (*Calvatia cyathiformis*) do have plump pedestals that smoothly flare up into a melon-shaped top. But all Puffballs have a very simple outline with no cap, no gills, no pores, no tentacles, no petals, no tutu, and no rings: just a whitish, asymmetric ball.

Because they come up when the weather is warm, they can go from zero to dusty maturity in less than a week. When you harvest other species of mushrooms, they are mature and have had a chance to spread spores (functionally, spores are akin to seeds). But when you harvest an immature, edible Puffball you are keeping it from reproducing. So don't harvest every Puffball you see—let some of them "go to seed," if you will. And then after dinner, go outside with the kids and kick a few mature Puffballs to make sure there will be more for next year.

FEASTING

These are tastier than store-bought mushrooms. Puffballs have a mild mushroom umami flavor and a texture not unlike tofu. Brush or cut off any dirt, as they absorb water too readily for rinsing. The skin is edible, so

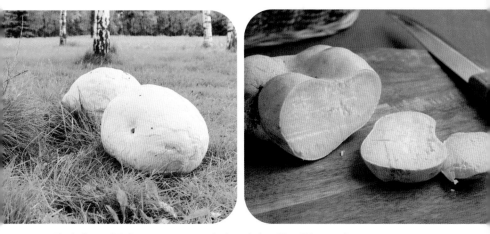

Thick slices of *Calvatia gigantea* can be breaded and fried like eggplant.

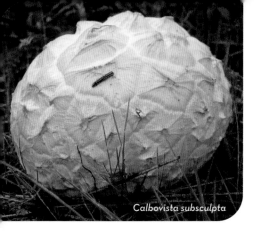

Calbovista subsculpta

small Puffballs can be eaten whole with eggs or tossed into a soup. For larger Puffballs, treat them like eggplant: Slice your specimen into ¼-inch-thick steaks, dip in egg, drag through seasoned flour or breadcrumbs, and fry in butter till crispy brown on the outside. Or dice into ½-inch cubes like home fries, sauté with garlic and seasonings, and serve as a side dish or tossed on a salad. "Wildman" Steve Brill's *The Wild Vegan Cookbook* has recipes for Puffballs in salads, marinara, lasagnas, and even a Puffball Parmesan.

PRESERVING

Puffballs stay fresh in a paper bag in the fridge for up to a week. If you have a surplus, slice into steaks and dry them at 100°F (38°C) until they are crisp as crackers. Save indefinitely in a glass jar. Pulverize in a blender for mushroom flour with which to flavor baked goods, make gravy, or coat cuts of meat.

FARMING

They are saprobes, living off decaying matter in the soil, but no one has cultivated them yet.

LOOK-ALIKES

It's a stretch, but immature egg forms of Amanitas and Stinkhorns can fool novices. Cut them open and the former show a mushroom outline and the latter a gelatinous alien-looking creature. Some may also mistake toxic *Scleroderma* mushrooms for Puffballs. But their skin is very tough and the interior flesh very dark.

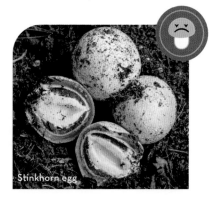

Stinkhorn egg

KNOW BEFORE YOU EAT

WHAT, WHERE & WHEN

- Saprobe that decomposes organic matter on the ground.

- Spore print, depending on species, may be yellow, greenish, brown, or purple. But if visible, the mushroom is too old to eat.

- Found in fields, lawns, meadows, and pastures growing from the ground.

- Sometimes found in woods with patches of grass (*Calvatia* species) or on very decomposed wood (*Lycoperdon* species).

- Found in the latter half of summer into fall in the Rockies and the East. From winter through spring on the West Coast.

FIELD ID CHECKLIST (ALL MUST BE CORRECT)

- Exterior: whitish skin. May be smooth or have pyramidal scales, warts, prongs, or hairs.

- Interior: soft and solid white from stem to stern, like tofu or a marshmallow. If you see other colors, gelatin, or an outline of a mushroom, toss it.

- Larger than a tennis ball: *Calbovista subsculpta* or *Calvatia* species sometimes as large as 5 feet across.

- Smaller than a tennis ball: *Lycoperdon* species sometimes as small as a marble.

NOTE: *This list can be used to ID all the species listed on page 142.*

KING BOLETE:
The Best Bolete to Eat

Boletus edulis

Meaning of the Latin name: Ancient Greek for "mushroom," edible

Also known as: *Cep* (France), *Steinpilz* (Germany), Penny Bun (United Kingdom), Porcini (Italy. *Porcinelli* is the common name Italians give to other, not-quite-so-delicious boletes that resemble porcini.)

Comparable species: Some mushroom hunters, including Michael Kuo and the late Gary Lincoff, consider the term "King Bolete" to encompass a number of closely related species, including *Boletus aereus, B. atkinsonii, B. barrowsii, B. clavipes, B. nobilissimus, B. pinicola, B. pinophilus, B. variipes, B. rubriceps,* as well as *B. edulis*. Whether or not they're related, all of these species are edible and do conform to the ID checklist on page 149.

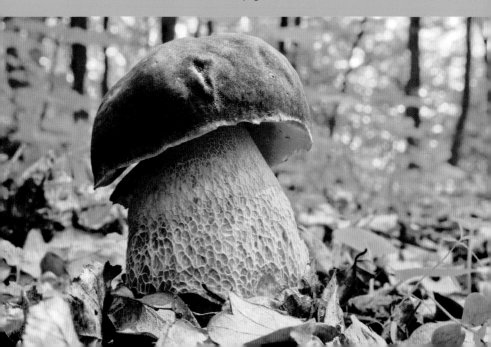

You don't get called the King for nothing. Handsome to look at. Great flavor. Dense texture. King Boletes are much sought after all over the United States and Canada, as well as much of Europe. Like other boletes, the flavor can be enhanced by dehydration. Which also makes them easier to share. But learn from my experience of being overenthusiastic in claiming a find as a King.

After poring over two keys online and one key in a mushroom book, I was pretty sure I had found my first King Bolete. It was young, small, and alone—characteristics that would incline me now to leave it be to produce more spores for the next generation. But novice foragers can be a greedy bunch. I sliced it up, sautéed it by itself in butter to better learn the flavor, and took my first bite. My eyes bugged out: It was horribly bitter. My first thought, "There must be something wrong with the butter." But the butter tasted fine. I went back to the keys and found I had overlooked something called Bitter Bolete. *Tylopilus felleus*. When young it looks like a King Bolete but the reticulation (netting) is brown, not white as with Kings. And if I'd waited overnight to do a spore print, I would have seen pink spores rather than the King's olive brown ones. After so much research, that bad taste in my mouth left me pretty crestfallen. And since common names are sort of up for grabs, I'd like

to christen this King Bolete look-alike, *Tylopilus felleus*, the Bummer Bolete. Lesson learned.

Even academic mycologists have a tough time correctly identifying many of the boletes (*Boletus, Leccinum, Tylopilus*, and more). They are a tricky bunch even with the best keys and lots of experience. So don't beat up on yourself if you have trouble moving beyond King Boletes and Old Man of the Woods (see page 153) in your first year or two. Many boletes are tasty, some are Sickeners. And some just look appetizing yet taste bitter. But the good ones are worth the effort.

FEASTING

This is a gourmet mushroom. With fresh specimens, the cap, sponge layer, and stalk should be cooked separately, due to differences in density and moisture (not the case with dehydrated

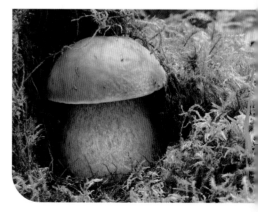

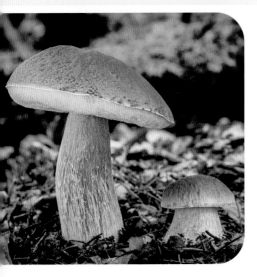

FARMING

It collaborates with the roots of trees, so has not been cultivated.

LOOK-ALIKES

Some bitter boletes resemble Kings, but a quick nibble will reveal that characteristic without having to make my mistake described above (although there are foragers who use bitter mushrooms to flavor their cocktails!).

There are boletes that are Sickeners, but none truly resemble the King Bolete, with one exception. The bellies of northeastern foragers have been plagued by *B. huronensis*, which resembles King Bolete and is sometimes called the False King Bolete. But *B. huronensis* has some key differences from Kings: It lacks reticulation and has yellow flesh that slowly stains blue.

boletes). To familiarize yourself with the flavor and texture, slice thin, dry-sauté, then add butter, garlic, and parsley. Goes well served with grains.

PRESERVING

Slice caps thin to dehydrate. Dehydration and rehydration improve the flavor (and sometimes the texture) of all edible boletes. When rehydrating, err on the side of soaking too little rather than too much—certainly less than 20 minutes. If using them in soups, stews, or sauces, it's not necessary to rehydrate—just toss them in.

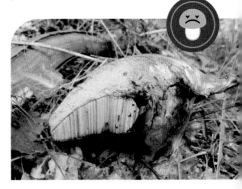

Boletus huronensis slowly stains blue when it's sliced open.

KNOW BEFORE YOU EAT

WHAT, WHERE & WHEN

- Mycorrhizal with tree roots.

- Yellow brown to olive brown spore print.

- Growing from the ground under conifers and deciduous trees.

- Scattered individuals and groups.

- Summer and fall in the East. Summer in the Rockies. Can occur in winter and spring in the West.

FIELD ID CHECKLIST (ALL MUST BE CORRECT)

- No cup, tutu, veil remnant, scales, or warts on cap or stalk.

- White to pale brown plump stalk, thicker and longer than your thumb.

- Plump cap is as wide or wider than your palm.

- Cap is yellow brown, brown, or reddish brown.

- Sponge layer under cap is white when young, becomes yellow, brown, or olive from spores when older.

- White interior flesh does not stain when cut.

- Fine, white reticulation (netting) on the upper portion of stalk.

- A nibble reveals no bitter taste.

NOTE: *This list can be used to ID the comparable species listed on page 146.*

Bummer Boletes:
Letdown City

It's true that boletes won't kill you. *But pursuing their mysterious identity can raise your blood pressure sometimes. At almost all stages of growth they can look appetizing in their form and color, but don't be deceived. After learning the King Bolete (page 146), the Old Man of the Woods (page 153), and a few other of the usually three to five local favorites, you will—like all of us—struggle to work your way through multiple keys, in multiple books and on multiple websites, to narrow down the identity of many a bolete. As the authors of the valuable and authoritative* North American Boletes: A Color Guide to the Fleshy Pored Mushrooms *say, "While some boletes are quite distinctive and easily recognized, others can be exceedingly difficult to identify, even for experienced boletologists."*

Did I say bolete? I also meant the many species that are discussed as being part of what are broadly considered to be boletes: Tylopilus, Suillus, Leccinum, Strobilomyces, Xanthoconium, *and nearly a dozen other genera. Sigh.*

But there is hope.

For decades foragers believed we had three quick tests we could apply to a bolete in the hand to decide if it was likely inedible (although we also knew that we were ruling out some edibles for the sake of simplicity):

- *Many bolete Sickeners had red or orange pore layers (under the cap).*

- *All other bolete Sickeners with pore layers of any color would stain blue (slowly or quickly) when touched or cut.*

- Any boletes that survived those two tests yet were too bitter to eat could be determined by tucking a little pinch of the flesh into the front of your mouth to chew for 10 to 15 seconds to see if it was mild or bitter, then spitting it out.

We thought that if your find survived all three of those tests, you could gather its comrades up and bring them home with confidence that they were all edible even if you didn't know the species.

But the forager grapevine slowly accumulated the various Sickeners that could be exceptions to those three rules: some with orange caps, some with scabers (a rough surface) on the stalks, and various species that didn't easily fall into categories.

But, as I said, there is hope.

The good foragers in the Western Pennsylvania Mushroom Club have put together a website called the Bolete Filter (see Resources, page 240). Here you can scroll through pages of photos of boletes like a book of mugshots at the police station. Between that website and a copy of North American Boletes, you will be able to identify many (but possibly not all) of your bolete finds.

And the three rules above? While they're not as airtight as we thought they were, they still play a useful role in excluding a lot of the likely Sickener boletes out there. And you can definitely still avoid the bitter ones.

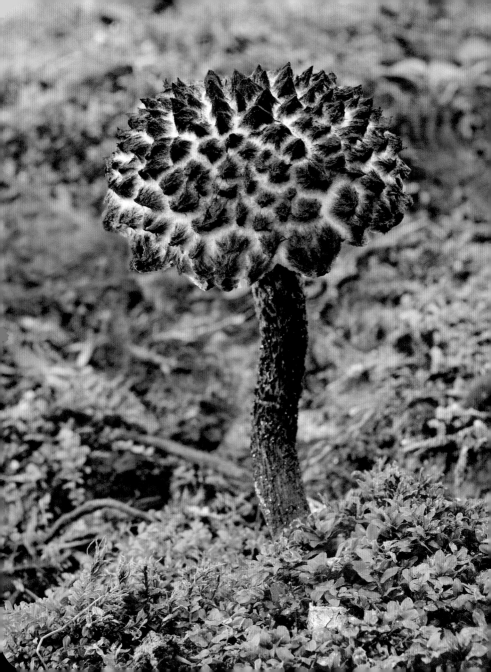

OLD MAN OF THE WOODS:
The Shroom That Needs a Shave

Strobilomyces strobilaceus

Meaning of the Latin name: pinecone, like a pinecone

Also known as: Pinecone Mushroom

Comparable species: *S. floccopus* (wooly), *S. dryophilus* (oak-loving), *S. confusus* (disorderly)

On one of my first forays, I heard another mushroom hunter say that he didn't harvest any mushrooms with gills, as some of those could kill you. So he only gathered mushrooms with pores under their caps, meaning polypores that grow on trees and boletes that grow on the ground.

I remember thinking that it might be true that only a gilled mushroom can kill you, but it seemed more productive to learn as many as you could, regardless of pores or gills.

Either way, that's the hunt on which I learned to identify the bolete called Old Man of the Woods. It's one of the easiest mushrooms for a novice to learn: It's distinct and has no look-alikes. I think the name comes from the image of an old man who's been retired

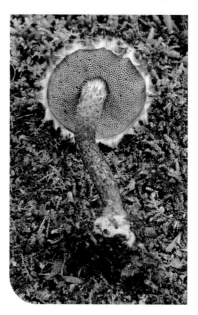

The cap resembles the bottom of a pinecone.

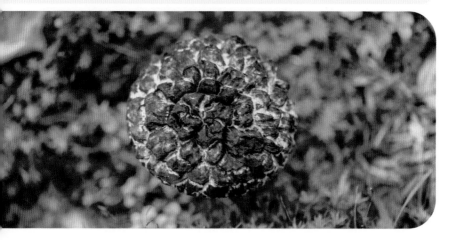

long enough to forgo the ritual daily shave. The entire cap is covered by blackish scales that resemble a grizzled beard. But you can also see that the cap resembles the bottom of a pine-cone, which explains the Latin name. To save some time and space, I'll refer to it as OMW from now on.

FEASTING

These are better than store-bought mushrooms. Some mushroom hunters like to peel off the pore layer and the stem before cooking, but on young ones they both taste fine to me. The texture of the stalk may be too tough for some. Slice the cap and dry-sauté if damp. Add butter, garlic, and a dash of salt. Note that OMW can stain a pot of food dark or black.

PRESERVING

OMW, like other boletes, is always improved by dehydrating. Slice and run through a dehydrator at 100°F (38°C) or lower overnight. Store in a jar in a dark place for up to a year or more. Rehydrate on the counter in water, milk, or wine until tender, or up to about 20 minutes. Save the flavorful soaking water for cooking rice, or add to soups and sauces.

FARMING

As mycorrhizal mushrooms they collaborate with tree roots, so they have not been cultivated.

LOOK-ALIKES

None.

WHAT, WHERE & WHEN

- Mycorrhizal with deciduous trees.

- Black to dark brown spore print.

- On the ground, in forests, under deciduous trees.

- Single or sometimes scattered.

- Eastern North America, but reportedly also in the Southwest.

- Late summer to early fall.

ID CHECKLIST (ALL MUST BE CORRECT)

- Cap *completely* covered by wooly, blackish scales: resembles the bottom of a pinecone.

- Underside of cap is spongelike.

- Underside of cap starts white but becomes gray, brown, or black.

- Cap more or less the size of your palm, stalk as long as your fingers.

- White flesh stains pink before darkening.

NOTE: *This list can be used to ID the comparable species listed on page 153.*

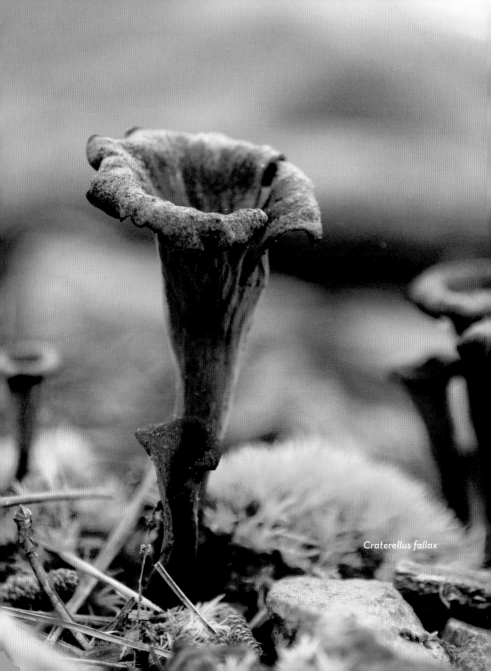

Craterellus fallax

BLACK TRUMPET:
The Fungal Telescope
Craterellus species

Meaning of the Latin name: volcano-like

Also known as: Horn of Plenty, Black Chanterelle, Trumpet of Death

Comparable species: C. *cornucopioides* (horn of plenty), C. *fallax* (deceptive), C. *foetidus* (smells bad), C. *cinereus* (gray)

There are no invisible mushrooms, but there is one you can see through: the Black Trumpet. They are about the size of a finger and grow in groups (like a disorderly brass band that refuses to shine their instruments), often in patches of moss. Like a trumpet, the bottom is narrow, the middle is a tube, and the top is flared open. They could also fairly be called black telescopes: Cut one off just above ground level and hold it to your eye. It's hollow. You'll be able to see through it, like a trumpet or a telescope.

It's uncertain if they have some affiliation with moss or if the ones growing in moss are just that much easier to spot. Their dark color makes them hard to see otherwise. An object is dark because it reflects little light. So dark things like Black Trumpets aren't eye-catching until you get

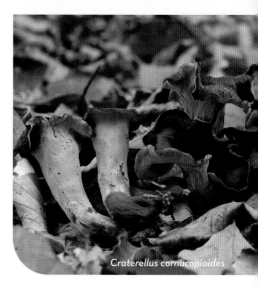

Craterellus cornucopioides

pretty close. And the contrast with the brighter, green mosses makes them visually pop out.

Black Trumpet isn't invisible, but you can see right through it.

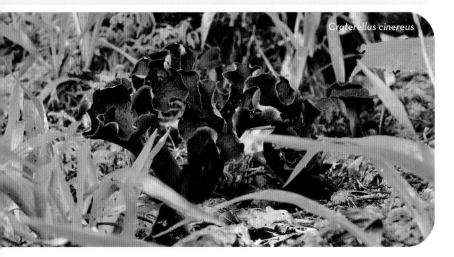

Craterellus cinereus

FEASTING

This flavorful, gourmet mushroom can be sautéed in butter with a little garlic and a dash of salt. The dark color nicely sets off lighter-colored dishes of eggs, grains, or fish.

PRESERVING

Only freeze if you've sautéed them in butter first. Doesn't respond well to pickling. Drying enhances the flavor. Dried Trumpets can be crumbled and added straight to soups, stews, or sauces for flavor. Or rehydrate and sauté and sprinkle onto dishes for flavor and color.

FARMING

Collaborates with tree roots, so has not been cultivated.

LOOK-ALIKES

Only other edible members of the genus really. But some foragers do try to confuse Black Trumpets with Devil's Urn (see page 68), which can be a similar size and mostly black. But Devil's Urn doesn't grow on the ground: It's found on sticks. Also, once you cut the stem of Devil's Urn, it looks like a bowl with a hole in the bottom, not a telescope. Lastly, the Black Trumpet fruits in late summer or fall while the Devil's Urn fruits in spring. There's no good reason to confuse them. Fortunately, they are both edible.

WHAT, WHERE & WHEN

- Mycorrhizal with tree roots.

- White, yellow, or pinkish yellow spore print.

- In deciduous woods on the forest floor.

- Found among moss most often. Unclear whether they favor growing with moss or if the moss merely makes Black Trumpets more visible.

- Summer and fall in the East. Fall and winter in the West.

FIELD ID CHECKLIST (ALL MUST BE CORRECT)

- No cup, tutu, veil remnant, scales, or warts on cap or stalk.

- Entire mushroom about the size of your finger.

- Narrow at the base and center, wide opening at the top.

- Black to brownish gray in color.

- Exterior may be smooth, wrinkled, or veinlike, but no gills.

- Snip it at ground level and hold it like a telescope. You can see through the length of the mushroom.

NOTE: *This list can be used to ID the comparable species listed on page 157.*

SHRIMP OF THE WOODS:
The Powdered Donut Fungus
Entoloma abortivum

Meaning of the Latin name: in-rolled margin, aborted

Also known as: Aborted Entoloma, Powdered Donut Mushroom, Powdered Donut of the Woods

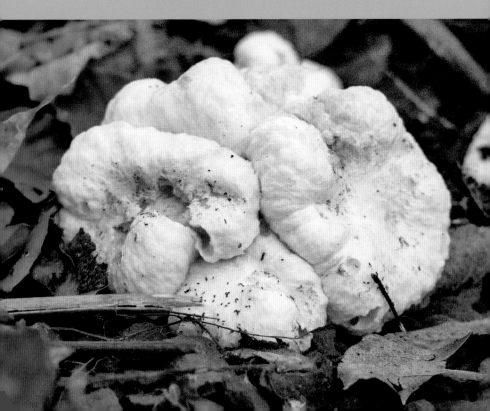

If you're trolling the forest hoping to net a few Shrimp of the Woods, you will be perplexed when you find them for the first time. These delicious mushrooms don't really look like shrimp until you've cleaned them up and they're sizzling in the skillet. Only then does its resemblance to the meaty body of a shrimp become evident.

I briefly worked on a shrimp boat as a young man, sorting hundreds of pounds of those crustaceans. But in the woods, these mushrooms have not looked like any shrimp I'd ever seen. The first time I saw this fungus, a colleague pointed out that they looked more like wrinkly powdered donuts someone had spilled on the ground.

The bottom line is that their odd shape and coating won't resemble any other mushroom you've seen. But what are these strange-looking creatures really?

They are actually two mushrooms in one. The underlying fungus is the Ringed Honey Mushroom (*Armillaria mellea*; see page 122). In an ironic case of ecological justice, Honey Mushrooms, which parasitize and kill deciduous trees, can themselves be parasitized by Shrimp of the Woods. This not only improves the flavor of the Honey Mushroom but also makes it unlikely to give you the kind of gastrointestinal distress that Honeys provoke in some people.

And it turns out the confusing common name isn't the only issue. Mycologists initially thought that the Honey Mushroom's mycelia attacked Shrimp of the Woods, causing it to abort and lose its mature form. But nature fooled the mycologists. It's the Shrimps that are attacking the Honeys and causing them to abort and lose their mature parasol shape.

The Shrimp of the Woods invades the Honey Mushroom with its mycelium until it no longer resembles a Honey Mushroom. The tissues thicken and become wrinkled. The cap and stem contort in upon themselves like a donut with a barely visible hole. The exterior becomes coated with a thin white layer resembling powdered sugar. A patch of them looks like a delivery-fail, courtesy of Krispy Kreme.

FEASTING

This is gourmet fare when well cooked. Convolutions in the mushroom can hold moisture, so there may be brown rotten spots that need to be cut away. Undercooked specimens have given this mushroom an undeservedly poor reputation. Dry-sauté to reduce moisture. Then add butter and continue to sauté until browned and reduced in size by about half. Add salt and/or garlic to taste. When well cooked, the texture is very good, and the flavor is mild and delicious.

These look like shrimp when they're sizzling in the skillet.

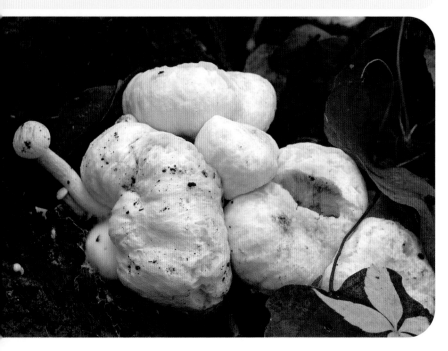

PRESERVING

Best preserved by being lightly sautéed and then frozen. Don't thaw. Just drop in a hot skillet to finish cooking.

FARMING

As a parasitizing fungus on another fungus, it has not yet been propagated.

LOOK-ALIKES

If you guessed there are no poisonous look-alikes, you'd be right. But

Shrimp of the Woods is not the same as another edible mushroom that goes by the name Shrimp Russula (*Russula xerampelina*). That one does not look like a shrimp at any stage. But some say it smells like shrimp or crab. That seems like one more reason to call *E. abortivum* "Powdered Donut Mushroom" instead. Why confuse beginners by duplicating mushroom common names?

WHAT, WHERE & WHEN

- *E. abortivum* is a parasite of *Armillaria* species, which are parasites of deciduous trees.

- Under deciduous trees. Found on the ground mostly in fused clusters. On or near decaying wood.

- May be near uninfected Honey Mushrooms (*Armillaria* species). Also, may be near mature *Entoloma* species, with gray caps and stalk, that are parasitizing the Honey Mushrooms. But these are not recommended for eating by novices, as other *Entoloma* species are very similar looking and poisonous.

- May have a hint of pink spores from nearby mature *Entoloma* species.

- East of the Rocky Mountains.

- Seen from late summer to midwinter in southern latitudes. Found in autumn in northern areas.

FIELD ID CHECKLIST (ALL MUST BE CORRECT)

- Individual specimens will fit in your palm.

- Cap has a convoluted shape like a powdered donut. Or vaguely like a brain.

- Missing or minimal stem.

- With rare exceptions, there are no visible gills; and those will be succumbing to the white coating covering the rest of the mushroom.

- Fibrous to scaly surface with a dull white color that can be rubbed off, revealing a pale pink to pale tan color.

- Interior looks marbled.

Big Night
(and Day) in Tuscany

The elderly Tuscan forager was giving me the eye. Literally. He had
one good eye and one glass eye from a youthful chainsaw accident.
His name was Severino. Then he bent down over my basket of mushrooms saying, "Si. Si. No. Si. No. No. Si. No."

Each "No" was punctuated with a flick of his wrist that sent my errant
mushrooms on an arc through the trees. Some mushrooms that look
familiar on one's own continent may turn out to be toxic on another.
A word to the wise.

Of course "Si" meant I had picked one of the many edible mushrooms our group would find that day: gallinacci (Chanterelles), porcinelli
(very good boletes, but not as good as a porcini), sanguinelli (Milk Caps
with orange "blood"), miniati (Purple Corals), dentini (Hedgehogs—
because of their teeth!), and ordinali. The last had brownish gray caps,
white gills, and a white stalk. I'm still not sure what species they were.

His safety check complete, he gave me the eye again, smiled, and
rattled off something I couldn't comprehend. I glanced at our host, a
local chestnut farmer named Luisa. She shrugged her shoulders and
smiled, too. Sometimes she did not understand Severino's southern
Tuscan dialect.

My wife, Chris, and I were celebrating our tenth anniversary by
spending the month of September in Italy. Our goal was to boat, bike,
stroll, and eat our way through Venice, Tuscany, and Umbria. Foraging
was a small part of our agenda, but it spawned some of our richest
stories from this trip. Foraging gives us the feeling of being a part of
nature, not just spectators. Here, foraging for fungi on Mount Amiata,

being a part of nature,

we felt like part of this forest of smooth sky-high beech trees and mossy boulders as big as houses.

Severino had spoken to me near the beginning of the foray: I had committed a fungal faux pas. I'd used my pocketknife to cut the stalk of a porcinello. I did it not to protect the mycelium; that notion has been disproven in several decades-long studies. But Severino dug out the base of the mushroom I'd left behind and dropped it in my basket. Dirt and all.

I didn't understand a word he'd said, but the sentiment was clear. Don't waste anything. He'd grown up in postwar rural poverty and had harvested mushrooms for his family's table since he was a boy. Foraging for mushrooms and wild, edible plants was important for survival in Italy until the economy started booming in the 1960s. But some modern Italians look down on foraging as a throwback to an earlier time of desperation.

We were lucky that Luisa knew Severino. He felt no shame about foraging. He still loved to be outdoors and was happy to share his knowledge with us. His grown son, Fulvio, came along and also knew many mushrooms. When nearby, he translated his father's commentary into modern Italian and then Luisa put it in English for my wife and me: "In the crevice under this boulder, Severino would sleep if it was too dark to go home. One fall the rains were late and the porcini didn't come."

When traveling, I defer to local knowledge as best I can. But this tossing of dirty mushrooms into a basket had me perplexed. As we continued gathering mushrooms, I pondered this question and came to a conclusion. When the person who cleans the mushrooms in the kitchen also gathers them, they tend to go in the basket clean. But perhaps in *a traditional culture where the man of the house hunts the mushrooms and the woman of the house cleans them . . .*

Back at Luisa's chestnut farm, I was the one cleaning the mushrooms. Despite claims to the contrary, mushrooms aren't harmed by a rinse under running water, so cleaning them didn't take too long. And pushing them around in a dry pan on medium heat will drive off excess moisture, anyway. Then add fat and you're on your way to a memorable meal.

Soon I had a couple of cutting boards heaped up with the six edible mushroom species we'd found that day. Chris and Luisa prepared a simple soup according to directions provided by Severino: a base of sautéed onions, carrots, celery; a layer of mushrooms; a layer of garlic-smeared croutons; another layer of mushrooms; and a final layer of croutons covered with water and simmered for hours. I sautéed a flight of the four most interesting mushrooms in butter, garlic, and parsley. With each mushroom—gallinacci, dentini, miniati, and porcinelli—cooked separately and served simply, we could contrast and compare their flavors and textures like so many wine connoisseurs.

The other diners included Luisa's guest, Sabrina, a 30-year-old astrophysicist from the Marche region with angelic beauty and brains; Toby, a short, sturdy, English vintner working on a farm owned by a Dutch family; and his seasonal assistant and old friend, a tall, limber American named Jim, who normally lived in Scotland with his Australian wife. Got that?

We called his creative use of the language Jim-talian, as he invented Italian-sounding words for any he didn't rightly know.

Before tucking into the fungal feast, both Toby and Jim announced that they each had "an irrational fear of mushrooms." The two Anglo-phones then went on to describe the story each one had heard "from

"an irrational fear of mushrooms."

a friend who knew the mushroom expert." In both stories, from different continents, the "expert" had accidentally served his family poisonous mushrooms. In each story, the wife and children had all died, while the husband suffered greatly, only to survive and live on in guilt and shame.

What did I think? Not damn likely. Actual experts simply don't make those kinds of mistakes.

But given the menu—mushroom soup, pasta with mushrooms, and my flight of buttery mushrooms—Toby and Jim had little choice but to live dangerously. And flirtatiously. There were clear indications of budding love between Luisa and Toby. Jim, an army veteran and former ballroom dance teacher, alternated between hilarious and bawdy stories and twirling and dipping the women across the floor between courses. At one point Sabrina wrapped her arms across her stomach—but not from indigestion. She simply couldn't catch her breath after one of Jim's hard-to-believe-but-I-guess-that-could-be-true stories.

Between the candlelight, laughter, long looks, tasty bites, and deep dips, I was frequently tempted to grab my camera. But I resisted. Being a participant still outweighed anything gained by becoming a spectator. Do you recall the eating, drinking, joking, and dancing scenes in Stanley Tucci's Italian restaurant from the movie Big Night? Well, this was our Big Night. No interruptions. No time-outs. All food and feelings until late.

During a moment that was quiet except for some chuckling and hard breathing after a laugh or a dance, Toby lit up, leaned over the table and asked, "Are there any dentini left?"

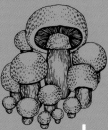

mushrooms
with gills
that grow on the ground

Gilled mushrooms on the ground are more common than other types of mushrooms. They do contain Killers among them, but careful comparisons of a few features will keep you safe.

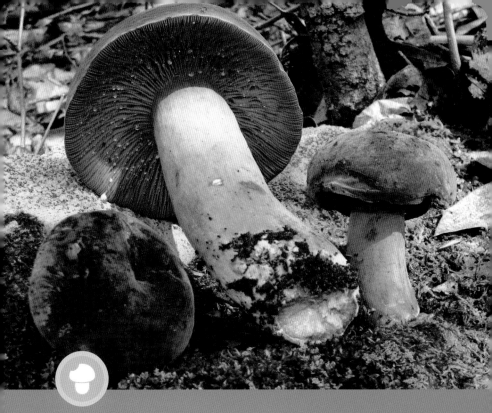

CORRUGATED MILKY: Looks Milky, Tastes Meaty

Lactarius corrugis

Meaning of the Latin name: pertaining to milk, having folds or wrinkles

Also known as: Wrinkled Milk Cap

Comparable species: *L. volemus* (exudes enough milk to fill the palm of the hand), known as Weeping Milk Cap, Leatherback Lactarius, or Tawny Milk Cap

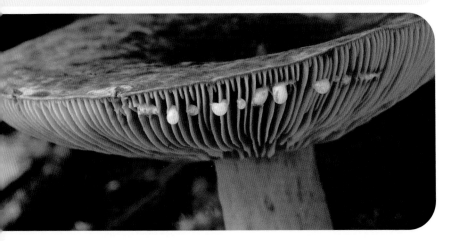

The first *Lactarius* species I learned was the Corrugated Milky. Seeing the latex flow from the brown-stained gills was magical. And I could say the same for that first taste of this mighty, meaty mushroom. *L. corrugis* and *L. volemus* are sometimes collectively called Fishcap Milkies or Golden Milkies.

I normally discourage using smell as an ID characteristic, because mushroom fragrance can vary and not all forager noses detect the same notes. But the fishiness of *L. volemus* (ditto with older *L. corrugis)* can be quite distinct. But don't forgo going through the rest of the ID list.

FEASTING

Sauté this gourmet mushroom for 5 to 10 minutes. Some say this is the meatiest of mushrooms.

It's advised to wear gloves when handling *L. volemus* to avoid smells and stains that can stick to your hands. Cooking dissipates the fishy smell of *L. volemus*.

PRESERVING

Sauté then freeze. Don't thaw them out—throw them straight into the hot pan.

FARMING

As mycorrhizal mushrooms they collaborate with tree roots and have not been cultivated.

LOOK-ALIKES

L. hygrophoroides looks very similar and is edible, but does not stain brown. Other Milk Caps with nonstaining latex may be bitter or acrid tasting.

WHAT, WHERE & WHEN

- Mycorrhizal with hardwood tree roots.

- White spore print.

- Grows from the ground in groups in hardwood or mixed forests.

- May be single, scattered groups, or entire fleets.

- Found east of the Rockies, more common in the Southeast.

- Summer and early fall.

FIELD ID CHECKLIST (ALL MUST BE CORRECT)

- No cup, tutu, veil remnant, scales, or warts on cap or stalk.

- Damaged gills release white latex that stains brown.

- Cap is about the size of your palm.

- Cap surface is velvety, pale brown to dark brown and corrugated or wrinkled (*L. corrugis*).

- Cap surface is smooth, sometimes showing concentric circles, light to dark orange brown (*L. volemus*).

- Stalk length more or less about the same width as cap.

- Gills and stalk are pale brown (*L. corrugis*).

- Stalk lighter color than cap.

- Gills are white to pale yellow (*L. volemus*).

- Older specimens smell fishy (*L. corrugis*).

- Often smells fishy (*L. volemus*).

NOTE: *This list can be used to ID the comparable species listed on page 169.*

CHANTERELLES:
Delicious Mushrooms That *Don't* Glow in the Dark
Cantharellus cibarius

Meaning of the Latin name: goblet-shaped, relating to food

Comparable species: *C. lateritius* (smooth like a tile), *C. appalachiensis* (from Appalachian Mountains), *Cantharellus californicus* (from California)

Even when people declare they know nothing about mushrooms, there's one they almost always mention in the next breath: "Ever find any Chanterelles?" It's understandable: At full height Chanterelles are bright yellow, no bigger than a day-old chick and almost as cute.

A charming name, an egg-yolk color, the fragrance of apricots (sometimes), and a flavor described as spicy or nutty conspire to make these one of the most sought-after wild mushrooms. Foragers in the Pacific Northwest ship 5 million pounds a year to Germany alone.

These are no bigger than a day-old chick and almost as cute.

They are also one of the mushrooms most likely to get novice foragers into trouble. Years ago, a friend of mine, relying only on a photo in a foraging book, was sure he had found a patch of Chanterelles. A chef of his acquaintance was equally sure and offered to buy them. He declined, having committed himself to serving them as part of a romantic dinner for his wife. The mushrooms were delicious. The dinner was romantic. In fact, it led to a bonding experience for them both: the shared misery of many hours spent hugging the toilet. They weren't Chanterelles but Jack O'Lantern mushrooms.

This story illustrates four fundamental things.

- Books are helpful in your foraging education, but they should supplement—not replace—time spent with an experienced forager.

- While most (but not all) poisonous plants warn you off by tasting nasty, poisonous mushrooms can taste delicious.

- It isn't mushrooms themselves that are dangerous: They aren't jumping in your mouth or biting you like a snake. It's careless mushroom hunters who are dangerous.

- No matter how good that poisonous mushroom tasted, the eating is not worth the repeating.

Closely follow the comparison below and you can indeed cook Chants, enjoy a romantic dinner with your partner, and perhaps spend the next few hours doing something that does not involve a toilet.

FEASTING

These gourmet mushrooms have a lovely flavor and texture and are best enjoyed by sautéing and serving as a stand-alone side dish. If eaten raw, they can cause gastrointestinal distress.

PRESERVING

Best to sauté surplus Chants for 5 to 10 minutes and then freeze in cupcake tins in case you don't want to cook all of them at once later. Pop out frozen clumps and store in a freezer bag. Do not thaw before popping into a hot skillet. They are often unwisely preserved by drying. That makes the rehydrated texture leathery unless ground to a powder in a food processor.

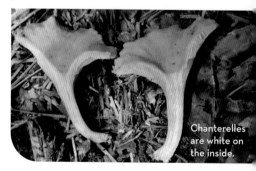

Chanterelles are white on the inside.

See Jack Glow

Gather the freshest caps of Jack O'Lanterns you can find. Wrap them in a damp paper towel and tuck them into a paper bag to preserve their moisture level. Go into the darkest space in your house, by which I mean no light at all. Perhaps an attic with no open vents or a closet with a rolled-up towel tucked at the base of the door to block light. You'll know it's dark enough if you find yourself blinking your eyes hard because you can't see a darn thing. In a couple of minutes your eyes will adjust and you should see the cap glowing a pale green light of bioluminescence (sadly, some Jacks won't glow). Do not die without witnessing this marvelous event at least once.

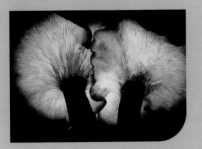

FARMING

Not yet cultivated, as it collaborates with tree roots.

LOOK-ALIKES

Jack O'Lanterns (*Omphalotus illudens* or *O. olivascens*) only vaguely resemble Chants, but eating these Sickeners is probably one of the most common mistakes made by novices. See details on sorting out the two below in the Field ID Checklist.

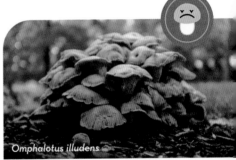

Omphalotus illudens

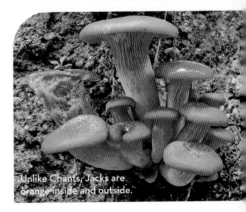

Unlike Chants, Jacks are orange inside and outside.

CHANTERELLES
KNOW BEFORE YOU EAT

WHAT, WHERE & WHEN

- Mycorrhizal with tree roots.

- White, yellow, or pink spore print.

- Scattered and in groups under trees.

- Summer and fall east of the Rockies. Fall, winter, and spring west of the Rockies.

FIELD ID CHECKLIST (ALL MUST BE CORRECT)

CHANTS	JACKS
Cap is up to the size of your palm, stalk may be as long as your fingers.	Cap is up to the size of your palm, stalk may be as long as your fingers.
Color varies from orangey yellow to clear yellow to a yellowish beige.	Consistently a pumpkin orange color.
White on the inside when cut open.	Just as orange on the inside as on the outside.
Coming from the ground as individual mushrooms.	Mushrooms grow fused at the base like a bouquet.
Very shallow gills that meander making V- and X-shaped crosses.	Deep, straight, parallel gills that don't fork or cross.

NOTE: *This list can be used to ID the comparable species listed on page 172.*

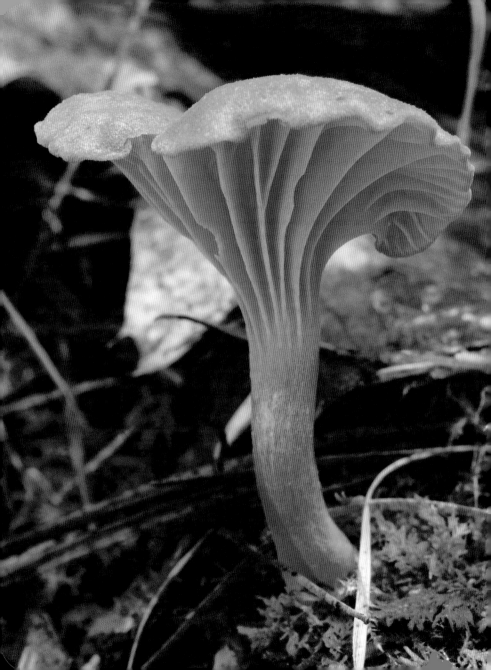

CINNABAR:
Looking Down So Far
Cantharellus cinnabarinus

Meaning of the Latin name: goblet-shaped, red pigment

Also known as: Cinnabar-Red Chanterelle, Red Chanterelle

The bright colors of Cinnabars will catch your eye from a distance and lift your spirits. No wonder they're considered by many to be one of the prettiest mushrooms in the woods. But their small numbers and tiny size means you won't be making many meals from them. Some foragers make the most of their color by pickling them or sautéing them to use as a garnish.

FEASTING

These are better than store-bought mushrooms. Their small size makes them quick to sauté. You can also toss them straight into soups.

PRESERVING

Cinnabars are rarely plentiful. And like other Chanterelles they don't dry well—they can be leathery when rehydrated. If plentiful, best to sauté and then freeze. Don't defrost. Just throw them straight into a hot skillet.

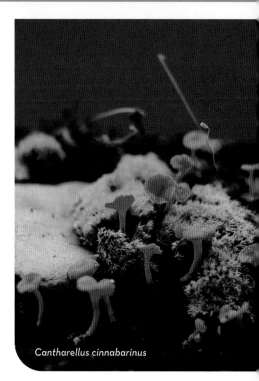

Cantharellus cinnabarinus

FARMING

Not yet cultivated, as it collaborates with tree roots.

LOOK-ALIKES

Some *Hygrocybe* and *Hygrophorus* species look sort of similar, but have waxy flesh or a slimy top and true, deep gills.

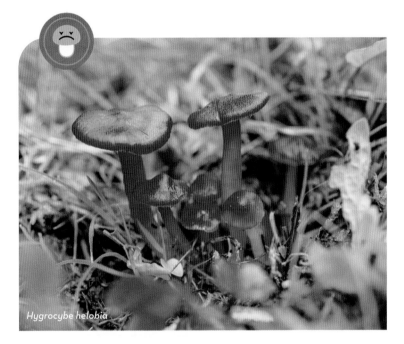

Hygrocybe helobia

WHAT, WHERE & WHEN

- Mycorrhizal with tree roots.

- Whitish to pinkish cream spore print.

- Found on the ground in hardwood forests.

- Small numbers in small groups but occasionally in large numbers.

- Common in eastern North America. Reportedly occurs in Arizona and the Pacific Northwest.

- Summer and early fall.

FIELD ID CHECKLIST (ALL MUST BE CORRECT)

- No cup, tutu, veil remnant, scales, or warts on cap or stalk.

- Striking flamingo pink to bright red or a reddish orange color all over.

- Interior may be whitish or tinged with cap color.

- Cap about the size of your thumb.

- Stalk slender and may be same or slightly longer than cap is wide.

- What appear at first to be gills are ridges that cross and fork.

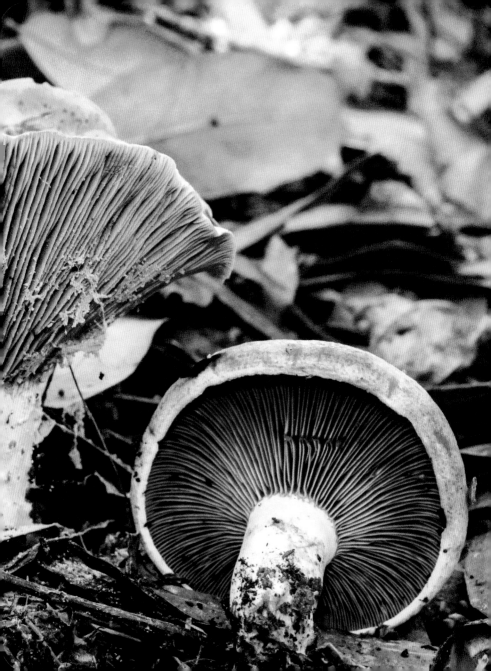

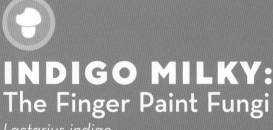

INDIGO MILKY:
The Finger Paint Fungi

Lactarius indigo

Meaning of the Latin name: pertaining to milk, blue

Also known as: Blue Milky, Indigo Milk Cap

I'm sure the picture of the blue-faced girl surprised some of the people who saw it posted on our North Carolina Mushroom Group on Facebook. She wasn't sick. She'd let her father smear the blue "milk" from this mushroom all over her face for laughs.

These are among the easiest of mushrooms for novices to identify. There are no poisonous look-alikes that will paint your fingers—or your face—blue.

As you might guess from the genus—*Lactarius*—these Indigos are part of a group of mushrooms that, when cut, release a small amount of milky fluid. Some of the others have white milk or orange milk. None of the not-blue Milk Caps will kill you, but a very small number of them can make you sick, and a few of them are shockingly bitter. In fact, it's rather a rite of passage for experienced foragers to invite novices to taste a bit of the white milk from the Pepper Milky (*L. piperatus*). The acrid flavor stings their tongue, makes their eyes pop open, and creates a long-lasting memory of watching fellow foragers cracking up.

FEASTING

These are better than store-bought mushrooms. Dry-sauté them first. When the amount of steam coming off the mushrooms has fallen significantly—just a few minutes—dial down the heat and add butter, ghee, or bacon fat and sauté for 5 to 10 minutes, or until the edges start to crisp up. This technique works well for any moist mushroom.

Are you a Dr. Seuss fan? Add some scrambled eggs; your Indigo Milkies will turn them green. But perhaps forgo the green ham. Young Indigos are delicious, but older ones can become bitter, contributing to mixed reviews of this worthwhile mushroom.

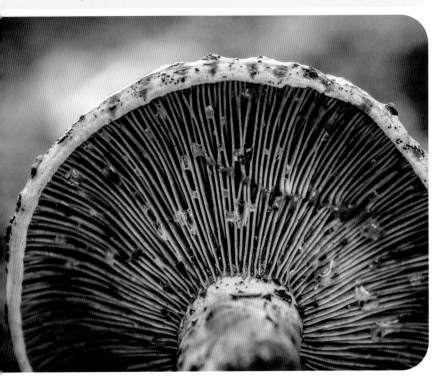

PRESERVING

Sauté and freeze. Don't thaw out—
throw them straight into a hot pan.

FARMING

It's mycorrhizal, so not yet cultivated.

LOOK-ALIKES

None really. Other bluish mushrooms
don't have milk or have milk of
a different color.

KNOW BEFORE YOU EAT

WHAT, WHERE & WHEN

- Mycorrhizal with the roots of conifers and deciduous trees.

- White to yellowish spore print.

- Growing on the ground in the woods as individuals or small groups.

- Common east of the Rockies and especially in the Southeast. Also reported in southwestern states.

- Midsummer into fall.

FIELD ID CHECKLIST (ALL MUST BE CORRECT)

- No cup, tutu, veil remnant, scales, or warts on cap or stalk.

- Cap, gills, stalk, and flesh are all various shades of color similar to faded blue jeans.

- Cut flesh or gills release a milky blue liquid, which slowly stains greenish.

- Gilled cap may get as large as, or a bit larger than, your palm.

- Stalk shorter than cap is wide.

- It's in the Russulaceae family, so young stalks snap like chalk.

LOBSTER MUSHROOM:
Two-for-One Fungi
Hypomyces lactifluorum

Meaning of the Latin name: under mushroom, milk flowing

When you find a Lobster Mushroom, you're actually looking at two fungi: a host and its parasite. Slice one in half and you'll see what I mean. Lobster Mushrooms have a thin layer of bright orangey red color on the outside and a bright white interior; colors very similar to the crustacean it's named after. If you could sample the DNA, you'd find that the white part is either a Pepper Milky (*Lactarius piperatus*) or, more likely, the Short-Stemmed Russula (*Russula brevipes*). Neither of these is poisonous, but neither one is tasty (although some chefs

do use the Pepper Milky as a spice). But once Lobster Mushroom attacks, covers, contorts, and devours either of these, it transforms the flavor of unmarketable mushrooms into gourmet gems—to the delight of foragers.

Some folks like to suggest that the Lobster might parasitize and hide the identity of a poisonous mushroom and harm some unlucky forager. But after many decades of recorded eating of Lobster Mushrooms on this continent, the number of instances of poisoning by Lobster Mushrooms adds up to exactly zero. I think some foragers can

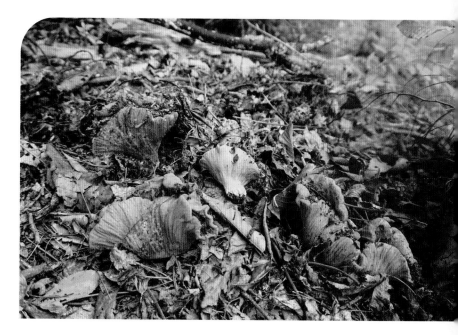

The reddish orange coating is another fungus entirely.

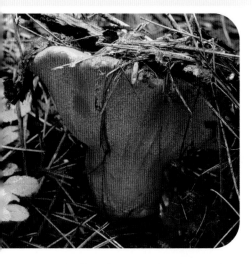

be like politicians in that they just like to tell scary stories, no matter how unfounded.

Lobster Mushrooms were among the first fungi I learned to identify on a mushroom walk. Like a weed coming up through a crack in the sidewalk, they sprouted right in the middle of a compacted footpath through the woods.

It's a truism among foragers that the best mushrooms are rarely found along a path—you have to go cross-country for the best finds. But in my experience, Lobsters like the compacted conditions of footpaths.

So why can they be found in paths? I'm not aware of any studies being done (the fungi industry has not invested nearly as much money in research as the fruit, vegetable, dairy, and meat industries), but I'll hazard a guess. The underground mycelia of the white mushrooms that come up in a path are stressed from the scarcity of oxygen in the compacted soil. That stress makes them more susceptible to pirate spores from Lobster Mushrooms that want to board the struggling mushrooms and seize their treasure. But if we foragers are on the right path at the right time, we can seize that treasure ourselves.

FEASTING

At their prime, Lobsters are sturdy enough to stand up to grilling after being brushed with a layer of cooking oil. They have a meaty texture even after a few minutes in a skillet. Definitely a gourmet mushroom!

PRESERVING

Dehydrate or cook then freeze.

FARMING

Being a parasite, it has not yet been farmed successfully.

LOOK-ALIKES

None.

KNOW BEFORE YOU EAT

WHAT, WHERE & WHEN

- A parasite that grows on *Lactarius* and *Russula* species, which are mycorrhizal on roots of deciduous and coniferous trees.

- On the ground, pushing up through forest duff. Sometimes in hard-packed paths.

- Often described as growing throughout the continent.

- Midsummer to mid-fall.

FIELD ID CHECKLIST (ALL MUST BE CORRECT)

- No cup, tutu, veil remnant, scales, or warts on cap or stalk.

- Bright orangey red color covers mushroom in a very thin layer.

- Bright white flesh (although sometimes pale yellowish).

- When the parasite is just getting started, there may be a "normal"-shaped mushroom cap. As the parasite spreads, the cap can be contorted into the look of a blown-out umbrella.

- Stem is shorter than your thumb.

- Cap size from smaller than your palm to as large as your outspread hand.

- Spore print not visible.

BLEWIT: A Colorful Treat on a Cold Day

Lepista nuda

Meaning of the Latin name: goblet, naked

Also known as: *Clitocybe nuda* (sloped head, naked), Wood Blewit, Bluefoot

Just when you think the weather is becoming too cold for nature to set the table, Blewits show up. Amid and sometimes under fallen tree leaves you'll find a little tribe of them, huddled together against the cold that turns their features blue. But they insulate themselves against the cold with a denser, meatier texture than similar-sized mushrooms. Expect to find them on warmer days after a frost. "Blewit" refers to the "blue hats" they wear when young.

This also might be the most challenging mushroom in this book for novices to accurately identify, as there are a few nasty look-alikes. The texture, flavor, and quantities of this mushroom make it worth including, but none of those things make it worth trying unless you're 100 percent certain. When in doubt, let the spores fall out. And forgo sampling any lacking violet color until you understand their characteristics thoroughly.

Don't hesitate to solicit opinions from more experienced mushroom hunters before preparing this (or any) mushroom for yourself or others. All these great flavors and textures pale mightily next to the guilt of sickening someone because you were in too much of a hurry to confirm a find or to wait to get a spore print.

FEASTING

Dry-sauté whole caps and stalks to remove excess moisture. Stir-fry with butter, garlic, and parsley until edges are crispy. Undercooked Blewits can cause gastrointestinal distress. Loses color after cooking. Tradd Cotter of Mushroom Mountain describes them as similar to "sweet and silky shiitakes."

PRESERVING

Best to freeze after cooking to preserve surplus. Can also be pickled, blanched, and preserved in oil or dried and ground for powder.

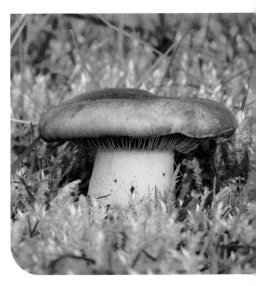

FARMING

Easily cultivated outdoors on wood chips or even cardboard.

LOOK-ALIKES

Some *Cortinarius* species, such as *C. violaceus*, are similar looking but will have a veil or veil remnant covering the gills and/or attached to the stem (like a tutu) and a rusty brown spore print. Some Corts are deadly poisonous. Some *Entoloma* species, such as *E. chalybaeum*, look similar and can be poisonous. They have a darker salmon-pinkish-brown spore print. *Laccaria amethystina* has purple gills, a long stalk, and a white spore print. Do not eat any of these look-alikes.

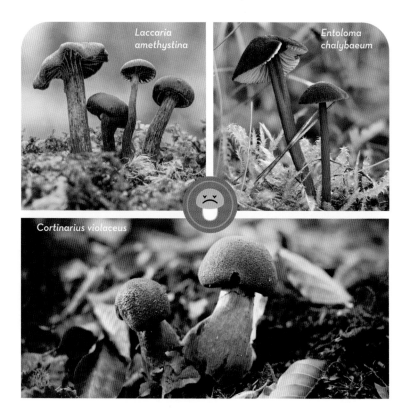

Laccaria amethystina

Entoloma chalybaeum

Cortinarius violaceus

KNOW BEFORE YOU EAT

WHAT, WHERE & WHEN

- Saprobe that devours organic matter in soil.

- On the ground. In deciduous or conifer forests, but also in mulch, compost piles, or fields.

- Occasionally solitary, but mostly in scattered groups.

- East of the Rockies, late fall into early winter. Triggered by freezing weather. May produce multiple crops per year. In the Rockies summer and fall. West of the Rockies in fall and winter.

FIELD ID CHECKLIST (ALL MUST BE CORRECT)

- No cup, tutu, veil remnant, scales, or warts on cap or stalk.

- Cap is the size of your palm or smaller.

- Caps of young ones have a distinctly rounded edge.

- Stalk is roughly the width of your thumb, but shorter. Mushroom looks short for the size of cap.

- The shape of young Blewits resembles that of store-bought button mushrooms.

- The bluish violet color will be visible on gills and/or stalk. Older specimens will exchange the bluish color for tan or pinkish tan. Variable in degree of color due to age or sunlight. Would be wise for novices to forgo any without the purplish color until better acquainted or get a spore print.

- Pale creamy pink to pinkish buff spore print. Novices advised to wait for a spore print on this species before eating.

steer clear of these killers and sickeners

It's important to know your enemies as well as you know your friends! Even though your goal is to learn to identify edible mushrooms, you'd do well to also learn the major Killers and Sickeners— so that you can avoid them. In addition to the mushrooms in this chapter, also see Jack O' Lantern (page 174) and Funeral Bells (page 128).

DEATH CAP
. . . or Dunce Cap?
Amanita phalloides

Meaning of the Latin name: named after Mount Amanus in Turkey, phallus

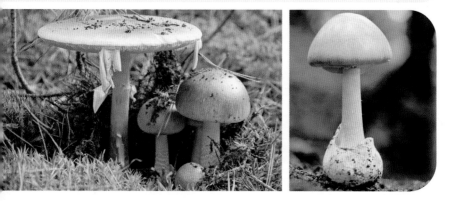

Most mushroom fatalities worldwide are from *Amanita* species. In 1965 a study in Europe revealed that of 109 people poisoned by Death Caps, 47 thought they were eating an edible species of *Russula*, which don't have veils, tutus, or grow from cups. Seventeen thought they were eating an edible *Agaricus* species. But they don't have white gills. And 45 thought they were eating an edible *Tricholoma* species, which have neither a veil nor a cup. This last point, especially, demonstrates the importance of digging up the base of an unfamiliar mushroom to rule out *Amanita* species.

Amatoxins will make you ill in 6 to 12 hours, but that will pass in a day, leaving you with the impression of suffering from mild food poisoning. But that's just the myco-calm before the fatal storm. Amatoxins will damage

dead in a few days unless you quickly get treated with silibinin—an extract from the milk thistle plant (*Silybum marianum*)—and an IV to sustain your salt and glucose levels. Some people's lives have been saved with a liver transplant, but you don't want to count on that.

LOOK-ALIKES

Best for novices to look askance at mushrooms with these features: (1) a tutu on the stalk and (2) the stalk nesting in a white cup. Other Amanitas have these features, but their caps may be a range of colors: white, yellow, green, tan, brown, orange, and red. Before breaking ground, Amanitas can be found in an egg form that some may mistake for an edible Puffball. Cut it open to reveal a mushroom profile. The egg later forms the cup and veil that

KNOW AND AVOID

WHAT, WHERE & WHEN

- Mycorrhizal with tree roots.
- White spore print.
- On the ground, under trees.
- Singles or a scattered few.
- Summer and fall east of the Rockies. Fall and winter in the West.

FIELD ID CHECKLIST (ALL MUST BE CORRECT)

- Cap is the size of your palm or larger. Stalk longer than cap is wide.
- White cup holding the base of the stalk.
- On young specimens, a white veil covers cap and gills.
- On mature specimens, veil has been ripped into a ring around the stalk (like a tutu) and sometimes shredded bits of the veil remain across cap.
- Cap color varies—greenish, yellowish, brownish.
- Gills and stalk are white.

DESTROYING ANGEL:
Anything but Heavenly
Amanita virosa complex

Meaning of the Latin name: named after Mount Amanus in Turkey, poisonous

Comparable species: *A. bisporigera* ("two-spored"—referring to the spore-bearing structure [called a "basidium"] inside the gills, which normally has four spores), *A. verna* (house servant), *A. ocreata* (shin guard—referring to the appearance of the volva)

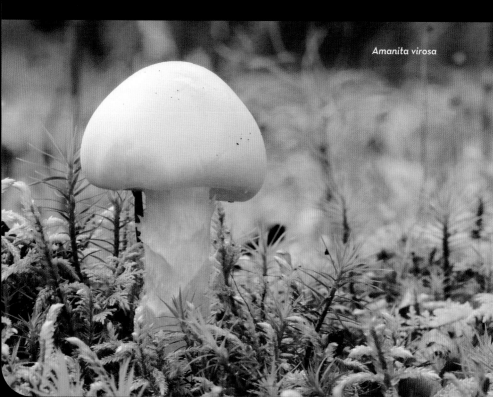

Amanita virosa

These "angels" are all white, like an angel on a Christmas tree. The first time you see one, it will be hard not to think, "That's so beautiful, it must be edible." But as a large number of mushroom hunters rehearsing to be stand-up comics have said, "They're all edible . . . once!"

Amanitas contain amatoxins. Within a day you'll think you ate a Sickener mushroom. Then you'll feel better and perhaps suspect it was just a bit of food poisoning from the factory-farmed meat in your dinner. Then, a few days later, once the amatoxin has moved from your bloodstream into your organs, your kidneys and liver will start to fail. Forty percent of patients die within a week.

Despite unfounded claims to the contrary, touching a poisonous mushroom or getting its spores on edible mushrooms will not harm anyone. The dosage of toxins in spores is way too small. But a few bites of the flesh are certainly fatal.

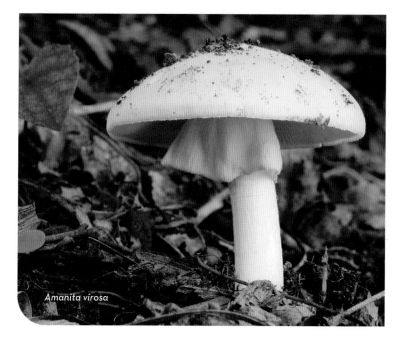

Amanita virosa

These "angels" are all white, like an angel on a Christmas tree.

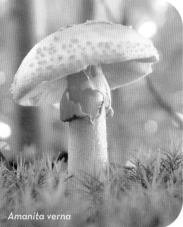

Amanita bisporigera

Amanita verna

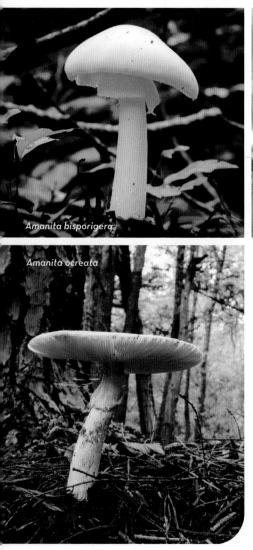

Amanita ocreata

Hopefully your doctor knows how to get their hands on some silibinin, an extract of milk thistle that counteracts the poison.

LOOK-ALIKES

Amanitas emerge from an egg form; at this stage, foragers may mistake it for an edible Puffball (see page 140). Cutting it open, however, will reveal the profile of a mushroom. Stinkhorns also form a white egg before they mature. Cut one open and you'll see a jellylike mushroom instead of the solid white of a Puffball.

DESTROYING ANGEL
KNOW AND AVOID

WHAT, WHERE & WHEN

- Mycorrhizal with conifers or deciduous trees.

- White spore print.

- On the ground under trees.

- Solitary or in scattered groups.

- Summer to fall east of the Rockies. Winter and spring west of the Rockies.

FIELD ID CHECKLIST (ALL MUST BE CORRECT)

- Mature cap bigger than your palm.

- Stalk as long or longer than cap is wide.

- Striking white cap, stalk, and gills. Rarely, may have hints of other colors on cap.

- Thick base nesting in dirty cup.

- While growing, the veil may be covering part or all of cap and/or gills.

- Veil remnant (like a tutu) around stalk when mature.

NOTE: *This list can be used to ID the comparable species listed on page 196.*

GREEN-SPORED PARASOL: It Will
Make You Green in the Gills

Chlorophyllum molybdites

Meaning of the Latin name: green gill, lead colored

Also known as: False Parasol, Green-Spored Lepiota, Vomiter

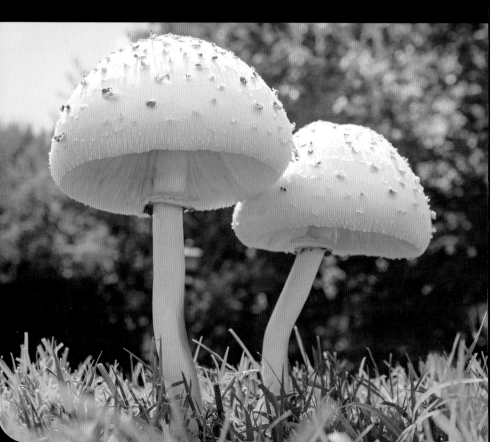

I always thought the phrase "you look a little green around the gills" to be odd. It implies that if you were a fish, you'd be sick and your gills would be green. But a fish's gills turn from pink to white when they are unwell. Once I learned about the Green-Spored Parasol, the likely meaning of the phrase became clear. When young, the gills are white and it looks uncomfortably like one of several edible fairy ring mushrooms. A too-enthusiastic mushroom hunter could certainly scoop some up, cook, and share them; they look, smell, and taste good. But only once.

Serving them at a dinner party will lead to a long, urgent line to the toilet. Onset of symptoms comes within a couple of hours. Symptoms pass in a day or two. Returning to the scene of the crime would reveal older Parasol mushrooms with greenish gills. This certainly happens often enough, as this is the most commonly eaten toxic mushroom in the United States and the single most common source of nonfatal poisonings. Reportedly, a small number of people have died from this mushroom.

Interestingly, a small number of people are resistant to this mushroom's toxin. And, of course, they'll want to share it. Another reason to be cautious with fairy ring mushrooms.

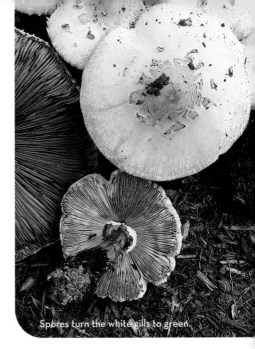
Spores turn the white gills to green.

LOOK-ALIKES

Some say there are about 60 species that reveal themselves in fairy rings. Many fairy ring mushrooms that resemble the Green-Spored Parasol are either a Sickener or a Killer: Even one Amanita is a look-alike of some fairy ring mushrooms. The Green-Spored Parasol is actually the poisonous look-alike for several edibles, such as the Horse Mushroom (*Agaricus arvensis*), Shaggy Parasol (*Lepiota rhacodes*), Parasol (*L. procera*), and Reddening Lepiota (*Leucoagaricus americanus*). None of these four have green gills

Accidentally serving them will lead your guests to form a long, urgent line to the toilet.

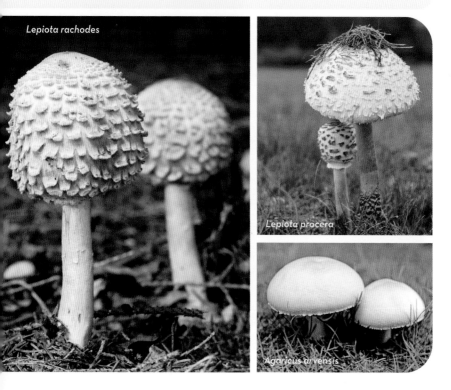

Lepiota rachodes

Lepiota procera

Agaricus arvensis

when mature (which begs the question, "Are you looking at mature samples?"). But not having green gills doesn't mean your fairy ring mushroom is safe to eat. They could just be young Green-Spored Parasols. Sorting these can be done with a very careful use of books and spore prints, but these species are best learned from a local expert.

Being able to identify the various fairy ring mushrooms and their look-alikes is definitely the sign of a skillful intermediate mushroom hunter. Novices should steer clear until they've been formally introduced by a knowledgeable local forager.

KNOW AND AVOID

WHAT, WHERE & WHEN

- Saprobe that decomposes organic matter in the soil.

- Lawns, fields, and pastures.

- Sage green to gray green spore print. Always check for the spore print with any fairy ring or similar mushrooms.

- Spring, summer, and fall in the Southeast. Summer and fall east of the Rockies. Summer in the Rockies and on the West Coast.

FIELD ID CHECKLIST (ALL MUST BE CORRECT)

- String of mushrooms in a lawn, field or pasture defining an arc or a very rough circle of any diameter. But sometimes alone or in scattered groups.

- When young, cap is closed and the mushroom vaguely resembles the shape and size of a chicken drumstick.

- When mature, cap may be as wide as your palm or wider than your open hand. Stalk is of a similar length to cap. Some caps can be dinner-plate size.

- Mature cap is white, but with a pale tan center and a smattering of tan scales.

- A veil covers the young gills, or is reduced to a loose tutu around the mature stalk.

- Stalk is white, but may have brown stains.

- Often when mature, cap and stalk remain mostly white, but gills become the sage green to gray green of the spores.

LITTLE BROWN MUSHROOM (LBM):
Not Worth Your Time

Minutus brunneus fungus

Meaning of the Latin name: Little Brown Mushrooms (I just made it up, actually)

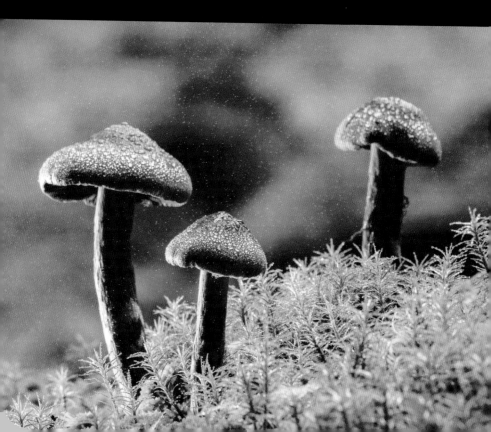

Even professional mycologists use the acronym Little Brown Mushroom (LBM) to describe the many hundreds of mushrooms out there that don't yield their secret identities very easily. The LBM you're looking at can be one of many species drawn from up to a dozen genera: *Collybia, Conocybe, Cortinarius, Entoloma, Galerina, Gymnopus, Inocybe, Marasmius, Mycena, Pholiota, Psathyrella,* or *Tubaria*. It's hard to say with certainty, but while most of these may well be edible-but-forgettable, others may also be regrettable. It's not worth the experimenting.

These species are often also responsible for what I call the 30-30-30 rule. Meaning that 30 minutes into your mushroom walk, you realize you've only gone 30 feet along the trail into the woods because the leader has stopped to identify 30 LBMs. If the leader is skillful enough to identify a few, they then have to answer the inevitable novice question, "Is it edible?"

Some LBMs will give you gastrointestinal distress, some of them will kill you, and very few of them are delicious, so the payback for time invested in cracking their code is very poor. Life is short (if lived well), so walk past these dull little gems of nature and focus your energy on larger, brighter, and more easily identified forest finds.

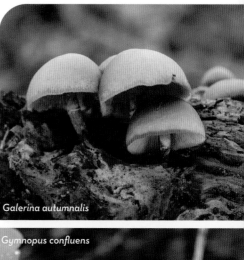

Galerina autumnalis

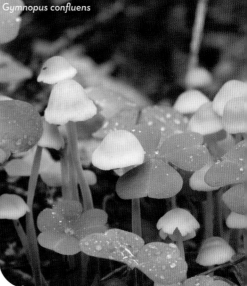

Gymnopus confluens

LOOK-ALIKES

Well, that's the problem isn't it? Funeral Bells (*Galerina autumnalis* or *G. marginata*), a.k.a. Tombstone Mushroom or Deadly Galerina, is a stalked mushroom with a small, brown cap that has the same toxins as the deadly Amanitas. Others, such as *Entoloma* species, can sicken you. Others are as yet undetermined in their edibility. Even professional mycologists struggle with little success to sort some of these species adequately, so why would you want to even try? If you see an LBM, just walk on by. Conserve your limited time on this Earth (and in the woods) for mushrooms that are less likely to be poisonous.

LITTLE BROWN MUSHROOMS
KNOW AND AVOID

WHAT, WHERE & WHEN
- Any season, any location.
- Spore print: really, who cares?!

FIELD ID CHECKLIST (ALL MUST BE CORRECT)
- Cap with gills, often no wider than a house key is long.
- Color: various shades of brown, but often dirty white, dirty yellow, or dull gray.

EMETIC RUSSULA: Red Alert!

Russula emetica group

Meaning of the Latin name: red, vomiting

Also known as: The Sickener, JAR (Just Another Russula), Brittle Gills

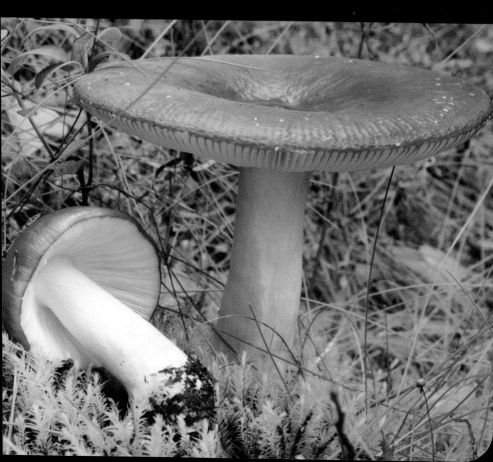

There are more than 100 species of red-capped Russulas worldwide.

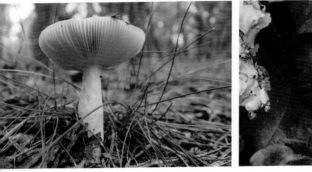
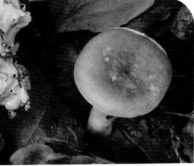

In many areas this appears to be one of the most common mushrooms. Then again, its bright red cap also makes it one of the most visible. For me, Russulas are memorable for being the mushrooms on which I learned an important mushroom ID characteristic. Stalks of fresh Russulas give a satisfying snap, like breaking a piece of chalk. Alternatively, you can throw them against a tree to watch them shatter (called the "shatter test," believe it or not). But I think stalk snapping is more reliable, as many fresh mushroom species also make a satisfying explosion on impact.

Not all red-capped Russulas are *R. emetica*, but at this point there's no good reason for an everyday mushroom hunter to try to sort them out, as you need a microscope to do so with many of them. Peter Roberts and Shelley Evans's *The Book of Fungi*, a handsome tome, says that there are more than 100 red-capped Russulas worldwide. And there's no reliable information that the other red-capped Russulas are any more edible or safe to eat. But they do shatter nicely.

As the specific epithet—*emetica*—implies, these will give you gastrointestinal distress. It has a red-hot taste with notes of acridity. It's reportedly edible after boiling, followed by salting or pickling. But I've never heard or read of a forager going to the trouble of doing that themselves outside of Russia and eastern Europe. I suspect that even after all that prep, *R. emetica* at best qualifies as edible-but-forgettable-if-not-downright-regrettable.

LOOK-ALIKES

Other red-capped Russulas, for which there is scant information about edibility.

EMETIC RUSSULA
KNOW AND AVOID

WHAT, WHERE & WHEN

- Mycorrhizal with conifers. Other red-capped Russulas collaborate with hardwoods.

- White spore print.

- Grows on the ground, in forests, singly or in groups.

- *R. emetica* and similar red-capped Russulas are found in winter in the West, summer in the Rockies, summer and fall in the East.

FIELD ID CHECKLIST (ALL MUST BE CORRECT)

- No cup, tutu, veil remnant, scales, or warts on cap or stalk.

- Stalks will snap like chalk (due to the presence of sphaerocysts). Older specimens don't snap so cleanly.

- Bright red cap fading to dark shades of pink.

- Cap is the size of your palm or smaller.

- Bright white gills and stalk.

- Stalk about as tall as cap is wide, and about as thick as a finger.

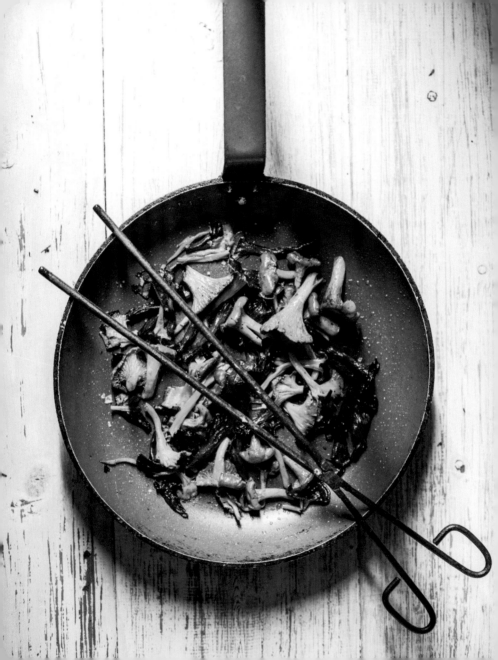

CHAPTER 5

COOKING & PRESERVING
Mushrooms

You don't have to be a chef to prepare gourmet mushrooms. You really don't have to be much of a cook at all. I'm proof of that. In fact, the less fuss made when cooking a new-to-you mushroom, the better you'll be able to register its flavors and textures. And preservation techniques for mushrooms are much simpler than canning fruits and vegetables. Mushrooms are gourmet foods that are easy to cook and easy to preserve. Becoming a forager is like winning an epicurean lottery.

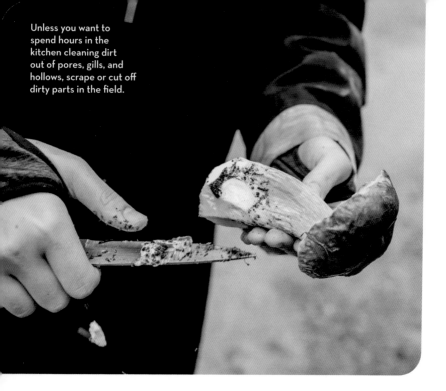

Unless you want to spend hours in the kitchen cleaning dirt out of pores, gills, and hollows, scrape or cut off dirty parts in the field.

CLEAN WHAT YOU GLEAN

Good mushroom prep starts in the field. When you go foraging, bring a sharp knife to cut the stem or base of a mushroom away from any part that's covered with dirt or infested with bugs. Carry a small paintbrush, shaving brush, or brife (see page 225) to flick dirt or bugs off the desirable part of the mushroom. The less dirt in the basket, the less will get stuck between gills and the less time you'll spend cleaning at home. Also, don't clean your mushrooms at the sink until you're ready to cook with them or preserve them.

STORE IN PAPER, NOT PLASTIC

If you're not cooking them right away, store them in paper bags rolled up tightly and park them in the crisper drawer. Depending on moisture level and species, they'll be fine for 3 to 10 days that way. Never put them in plastic bags; the moisture mushrooms transpire will condense and promote the growth of bad bacteria or fungi.

WASHING IS OKAY

Contrary to "common knowledge," you can wash mushrooms under the kitchen spigot. Kitchen authority Harold McGee disproved the notion that mushrooms absorb water long ago. But they will come with their own moisture level that slows down the cooking process. So a dry sauté (see Expert Tips for Cooking Mushrooms, page 216) will resolve that issue. Those that may have insects tucked away inside them, such as Morels and Egg Noodle Mushrooms, can be safely soaked in cold, salted water for 10 minutes, then rinsed and allowed to dry on paper towels or dry-sautéed.

Amazingly, Lion's Mane actually begs for a brisk shower under the spigot. After rinsing out any debris, twist this mushroom gently with both hands as if it were a sponge. Excess water will pour out. And I mean *pour*. Then the mushroom will return to its shape fully intact, as if it were a sponge. I have done this many times and have always been amazed at how much twisting pressure a fresh Lion's Mane can withstand. It makes me laugh.

Next, I hand-shred it to bite-size pieces so it looks like crabmeat. Then, depending on its moisture level, I may dry-sauté it before using it as a crab substitute in a crab cake recipe.

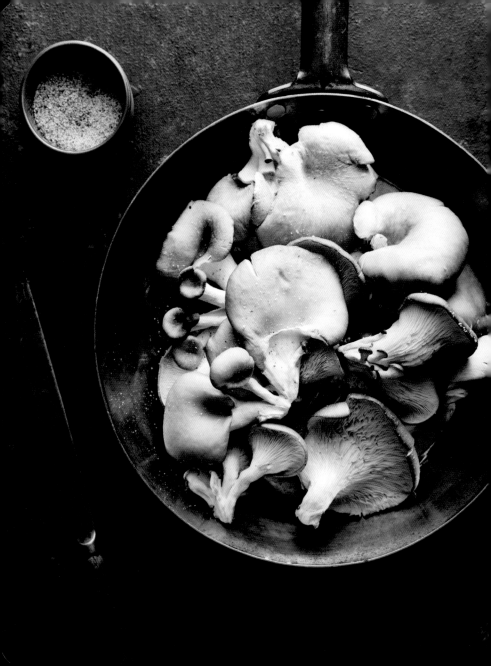

COOKING MUSHROOMS

I'm pretty sure you've eaten raw mushrooms bought from the store, but there are multiple reasons to cook them well first. Denaturing the toxins in edible mushrooms like Morels and Chanterelles is just one of those reasons. And as a novice, do err on the side of cooking a little bit too long rather than a little too short until you know if you or your family have any sensitivities to particular species.

As a general rule you don't *need* a mushroom-specific recipe. You can use mushrooms in any recipe in the same way you'd use cooked portions of meat: in soups and stews; in salads; as a side dish; as slabs on the grill or under the broiler; on pizza; and so on.

Interestingly, some mushrooms taste better when cooked in water rather than fat. But this doesn't seem to be a fully explored aspect of mushroom cookery to date. From Long Litt Woon's book *The Way Through the Woods: On Mushrooms and Mourning* I learned that when her Norwegian friends had cooked the very expensive Matsutake mushroom with butter, salt, and pepper, they weren't impressed with the flavor. She discovered that "mushrooms with a fat-soluble aroma are best cooked with butter, but the Matsutake's aroma is water-soluble, so this mushroom only really comes into its own when used in soup or rice. To make Japanese-style Matsutake rice, bring the rice to a boil, add a handful of chopped Matsutakes, turn down the heat, and cover with a lid. Then it's simply a matter of waiting for the flavor of the rice and mushrooms to blend and harmonize."

When learning how to cook a new-to-me mushroom, I often fork up a small taste to see how the flavor and texture are progressing as it's cooking.

Expert Tips for Cooking Mushrooms

The next mushroom book you buy *should be a copy of Chad Hyatt's* The Mushroom Hunter's Kitchen: Reimagining Comfort Food with a Chef Forager. *Regardless of your skills cooking meats and vegetables, you need this book to fully enjoy eating mushrooms.*

His interests in becoming a forager and becoming a chef developed at the same time—to our great benefit. Because their physiology is so different, mushrooms don't respond to cooking techniques the same way as animal- and plant-based food. Plus, a lot of the "common knowledge" about handling and cooking mushrooms is out-of-date. Most cookbooks would have you toss the mushrooms into the pan with fat and watch them simmer in their own watery juices, resistant to browning. I believe the resulting mushy texture is one of the things that has turned so many people into mushroom haters.

To brown mushrooms, Hyatt suggests instead a dry sauté for many mushrooms: "Get a heavy-bottomed skillet on a medium-high to high flame. When the [dry] pan is screaming hot, add the mushrooms and a pinch of salt and toss and stir the mushrooms regularly, until they start to release their moisture. As the liquid comes out and fills the pan, keep the heat high so that the water evaporates and reduces as quickly as possible."

With the moisture driven off, you can reduce the heat, add your cooking fat, and continue to sauté and season the mushrooms as desired. He learned this technique from mushroom expert David Arora. I learned it from Alan Muskat of the website No Taste Like Home, and

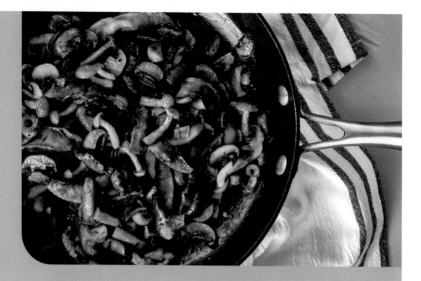

it has spread through the foraging community like beneficial mycelia. But this technique has not made the same penetration in restaurants and home kitchens that it deserves to.

If you're unsure about tossing mushrooms into a hot, dry pan, build your confidence by starting with the heat set on medium-low. And use a metal spatula with a straight edge, so you can keep the mushrooms from sticking to the pan. Watch the volume of water and steam that's driven off. When you notice that the volume has begun to decline, that's the time to add the cooking fat.

On another front, I had always avoided boiling mushrooms because it sounded like a way to turn them to mush. But I learned from Hyatt that because of their chitin, they retain their texture and, in some cases, become delightfully firm. For these and many other reasons, I strongly recommend that you make his book the next step on your foraging journey.

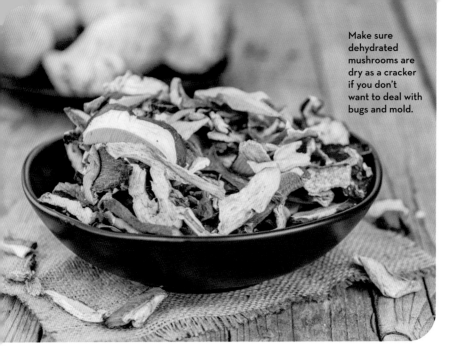

Make sure dehydrated mushrooms are dry as a cracker if you don't want to deal with bugs and mold.

PRESERVING MUSHROOMS

Freezing or dehydrating are your two best options for preserving mushrooms. Both techniques are very low-tech, and they sure beat letting a fungal surplus go to waste.

FREEZING

Most mushrooms can be sliced or hand-shredded, sautéed or braised in liquid for about 10 minutes, and then frozen in cupcake tins. Pop the shroomcakes into freezer bags; they'll store for up to 6 months in the freezer without losing their texture. Don't thaw them out before cooking—they'll get mushy. Just toss them directly into the hot skillet.

The only mushroom that seems to do well being frozen without being cooked first is Hen of the Woods (see page 96). I think Hens handle being frozen raw better than other mushrooms because their narrow season overlaps with the off-and-on first frosts of autumn. But I don't have any proof of that. After cleaning, I tear or cut each frond into a separate piece the size of a chicken wing or drumstick, then spread them out on a baking sheet and keep them in the freezer until frozen solid, about 20 to 30 minutes. As individual units, they can be popped into freezer bags and then removed as individuals rather than ungainly clumps. To cook them, I spread the still-frozen pieces in a casserole; cover them with oil, salt, and pepper; and cook for about 30 minutes at 400°F (200°C). At the 15-minute mark, I stir them around. They come out meaty, tasty, and ready for a dipping sauce.

DEHYDRATING AND REHYDRATING

A dehydrator is a great investment for a forager. The time will come when you have too many mushrooms to eat at once and you want to save them for another time. Or you want to preserve them in a way that doesn't take up valuable real estate in the freezer. Dehydration also provides an easy way to share them with friends.

After cleaning, slice the mushrooms into about ¼-inch-thick pieces and place them on dehydrator trays. Set the temperature at about 100°F (38°C) and let it run overnight. Don't be tempted to try to dehydrate your mushrooms in an oven! Some ovens won't go to a low enough temperature. Even the lowest oven temperature may cook the mushrooms, which is not what you want.

Check that the mushrooms are dry and crispy as crackers. If they are just leathery, there is still enough moisture to support mold and perhaps insects, so keep dehydrating them further. Once the mushroom slices are crispy, you can be sure that larvae will have fled and any eggs will have dried out. Load your crispy mushroom slices into clear jars and store them in dark cabinets. They should last indefinitely.

Some foragers also recommend freezing dried mushrooms to preclude any loss to bugs. In particular, Turkey Tails and Reishi sometimes contain larvae that survive the dehydrating process. So the additional step of freezing may be helpful there. But most foragers report no problems simply storing dried mushrooms in jars and without freezing. Dried mushrooms stored in plastic bags are vulnerable to insects that can chew through plastic.

There is a consensus that dried Black Trumpets and boletes taste even better than fresh samples. Something to consider.

A pound of fresh mushrooms dehydrates to about 3 ounces. When you're ready to cook your mushrooms, rehydrate in a bowl with water, wine, beer, stock, vinegar, cream, or milk. Depending on size, species, and type of liquid, they'll need 5 to 30 minutes to rehydrate, so monitor conditions. Overhydrated mushrooms become mushy. Save the liquid for cooking rice, flavoring soup, and other uses.

POWDERING

All mushrooms can be dehydrated, but not all retain a good texture on rehydration. Morels do well, for example, but Chanterelles do not—their texture becomes leathery. For such mushrooms, the alternative is to powder the dried mushrooms in a food processor. The resulting powder can flavor soups or coat cuts of meat, among numerous other uses. Sliced, dried, and powdered Puffballs, for example, make a flavorful addition to bread recipes.

Mycophobia Prescriptions

I've found three recipes that I recommend for bringing mycophobes and the myco-curious around. When I have Chicken of the Woods, I make a chicken salad dish, slap it in Tupperware, and bring it to gatherings. The more adventurous take a bite and go on about how much it tastes like chicken: "Is that really a mushroom?" Then the less adventurous are inspired to try it, and on down the spectrum of scaredy cats. It's a real conversion tool.

And for those who have a problem with the textures of mushrooms, I slice and sauté Oyster Mushrooms in bacon fat for 25 minutes. The deep gills become as crispy as fried chicken batter and the meaty caps become all porky tasting. Even my wife, who deeply dislikes mushroom textures, has been known to ask for seconds.

The third thing I've done is make a mini mushroom buffet of three or more species, each cooked separately in butter/garlic/salt/parsley and then set out for sampling. Knowing they have choices assures the myco-challenged that they may find at least one mushroom they can enjoy. It also makes it easy for experienced mycophagists to note the subtle differences in flavor and texture that get lost in more complex recipes.

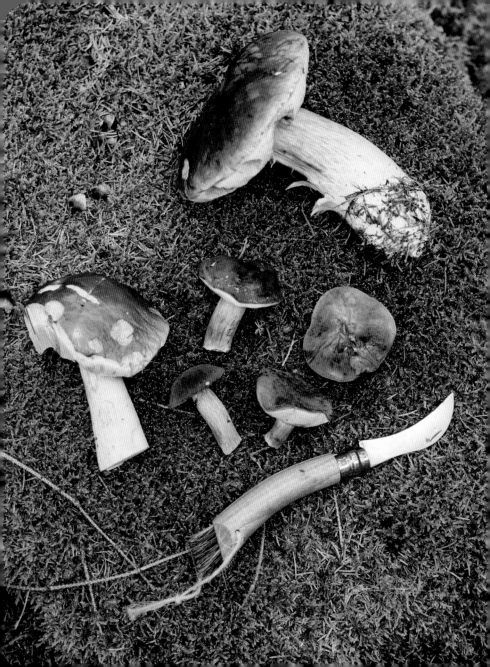

CHAPTER 6

Getting All
TOOLED UP

Having the right tools makes everything easier, whether its carpentry, stone masonry, or writing. With the right saws, chisels, or laptop, you can grow from success to success. Same goes for foraging.

YOUR TOOL WISH LIST

Here are the tools that will make your foraging life easier. You don't need to get all of them at once. You can fill your toolbox slowly. In fact, I suggest the way to go is to let the right folks know what you'd like in the way of a birthday present or a stocking stuffer. Beats getting another sweater with a reindeer on it.

FORAGING JOURNAL

Have one of these before you go on your first foray. You'll want to write down the little details that your expert shares. You'll also want to write down the date and location. A year or three later, you may not remember this spot. And having a journal that lists dates that you found different species helps you return in time to gather another crop. Don't worry that recording the location will offend your foray leader. They haven't taken you to any of their best spots!

POCKETKNIFE

I think everyone should carry a pocketknife whether they forage or not. I use mine at least once a day: opening mail, cutting open blister packs from the store, gathering flowers in the garden, and, of course, cutting mushrooms loose from their bed of soil or their harbor of wood.

There are plenty of good knives out there, but the brand I recommend is called Opinel. It's a French-made pocketknife produced in a variety of sizes. The handle is sustainably harvested French beech wood. In 1985, along with Rolex watches and the Porsche 911, it was declared one of the 100 best-designed objects in the world by the folks at the Victoria and Albert Museum. They are a thing of simplicity and beauty. And they are not expensive at all. Opinel makes a forager's knife with a brush included.

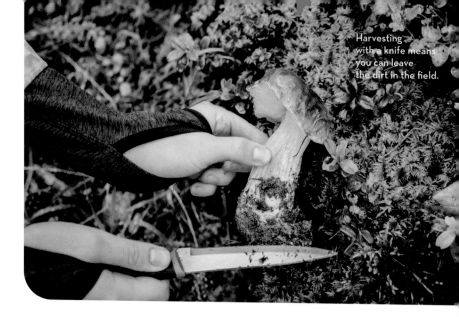

Harvesting with a knife means you can leave the dirt in the field.

Warning #1: Don't forget and take it on the plane with you. It will be confiscated. Warning #2: If the mushroom you're gathering is one you're not familiar with, don't cut it at ground level. Instead, use your fingers, a trowel, a hori-hori knife (details on page 226), or, last choice, your knife to dig up the base of the mushroom. Some poisonous mushrooms grow out of a cup or stacked rings, and sometimes you'll need to see this characteristic to get an accurate ID.

BRIFE

This is a brush with a knife. Opinel and other companies sell them for mushroom hunting. The reason you would want one is to keep dirt out of your basket or bag. First you cut the stalk just above the soil line. Then the brush lets you remove any debris: dirt, bugs, leaves. You may still need to do some washing when you get home, but on-site cleanup is an important time-saver.

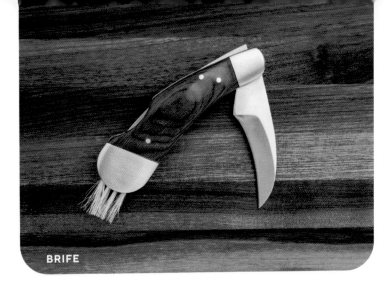

BRIFE

There are folks who think it's necessary to cut mushrooms rather than yank them from the soil to protect the underlying mycelium and promote more fruit in following years. Science shows us that isn't a concern. Three 30-year-long studies in Oregon, Germany, and Switzerland all confirmed that whether mushrooms were cut from the ground or yanked right out didn't diminish future harvests. In fact, yanking sometimes shows a slight increase in growth the following year. The advantage to cutting them is just that it reduces time spent cleaning them. But if you find a motherlode of mushrooms and you're knifeless (or worse—brifeless!), just yank away.

HORI-HORI KNIFE

This is sold as a garden tool, but it was invented a thousand years ago by mountain foragers in Japan. It's made for digging edible roots from soil that's rocky or dense with clay. It has a wooden handle and a thick, 6-inch blade that's over an inch wide. One side of the blade is serrated, and the other side is straight and sharp. It's a

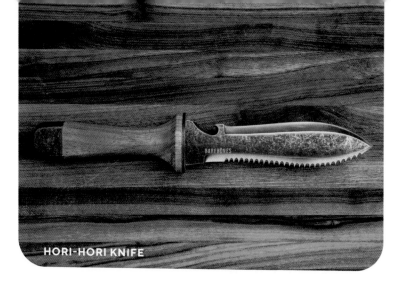

HORI-HORI KNIFE

great digging tool for gathering edible roots, truffles, or the base of mushrooms. I strongly advise mushroom foragers also to learn the wild edible plants you might run across. No sense passing up free gourmet food.

BASKET OR BAG

What will you carry your mushrooms in? Traditionally, people use baskets. They're lightweight, and the openings allow the spores of your mushrooms to drop out and onto new ground (kind of like Johnny Appleseed planting orchards across the countryside).

But many people find day packs to be more practical: You can travel hands-free over rough ground. And truth be told, by the time you harvest a mushroom it's already had enough time to spew billions of spores into the air.

Some foragers use mesh bags to gather mushrooms. They're lightweight, and spores can fall easily through the mesh. Plus you can show off your finds.

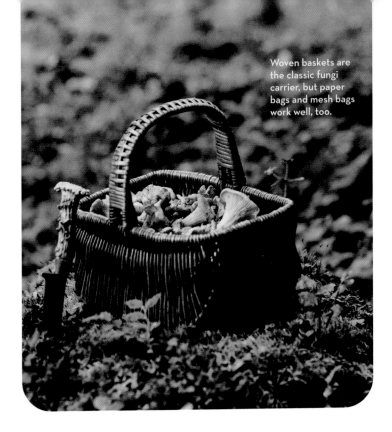

Woven baskets are the classic fungi carrier, but paper bags and mesh bags work well, too.

I split the difference. My sister made me a deep basket for holding wine bottles. I put a strap around the handle so I can loop it over my shoulder. It has gaps for spores to fall through and is deep enough to carry my tools, a water bottle, and even the occasional animal skull or tortoise shell I find in the woods.

PAPER BAGS OR WAX BAGS

To get your mushrooms home and to store them in the fridge, you'll want paper bags or wax bags. Plastic bags might sound convenient, but your mushrooms are breathing out moisture. As the moisture collects in your plastic bag, it promotes the growth of bacteria that can give you some gastrointestinal distress even if you cook them. Paper or wax bags are better; just fold the top over a couple of times and store them in the crisper section of your fridge so they don't dry out too fast.

POLE PRUNER

Gardeners use a pole pruner to remove branches from overhead. Some have an extendable pole that gives you a reach of up to about 12 feet or more. These are great when you find a Santa's Beard or Chicken of the Woods farther up a tree than you can reach. One concern: As you cut or pull on the mushroom, it will come loose and fall to the ground and break into pieces. It's still edible but dirty and sometimes shattered. Having a partner deft enough to catch it for you will really pay off.

FOLDING LADDER

I'm often out in my pickup truck when I see a delicious mushroom growing from a tree in someone's front yard. I always ask for permission to harvest it with an offer to share it with the homeowner. Ninety-five percent of the time, they make a face and say they're happy for me to have it and would I please come back each year to get rid of it for them. I put this information into my foraging journal.

Fall and winter are high season in North Carolina for treeborne mushrooms. So that's when I lay my folding ladder in the truck bed. Unlike an extension ladder, it is short enough to lay down flat in the bed. It is a little on the heavy side, so I don't recommend one unless you've got pretty good upper-body strength. But it will get you 20 feet high in a tree.

Captain Woody's Mushroom Hook

True, there are no old *and* bold mushroom hunters. *But that still leaves plenty of old mushroom hunters with their joints a-creaking as they squat to scoop up edible fungi in the fields. And the older we get, the less comfortable that squatting down or bending over becomes. But what if there were some way to bring those Chanterelles, Morels, and Milk Caps a bit closer? All without putting those older backs, hips, and knees through a mycologically induced stress test?*

Woody Collins has solved that problem by inventing a mushroom hook. From a standing position Woody—and foragers of any age who are handy enough to make a tool like his—can gather soilborne mushrooms quickly and with little or no dirt on them. A tool like this is also handy as a walking stick; for pushing leaves aside, holding brush back, and snagging treeborne mushrooms; and as an alternative to using your face to plow through spiderwebs.

Woody is what the young folks might call a "maker." Before he became a mushroom hunter, he spent 30 years on shrimp boats as mate and captain. As those who work in farming and fishing know, sometimes the budget isn't there to buy some dandy tool. So you have to make one yourself. And sometimes those tools are concocted with stunning creativity. Especially when you're several miles at sea.

Retired from shrimping, Woody now gathers many pounds of Chanterelles that he finds in the South Carolina Lowcountry's gothic forests of live oaks draped with Spanish moss. He's still plenty spry, but when he wanted a quicker way to get those mushrooms into his basket, he put his maker skills to work. He says he also wanted to avoid plunking down to pick mushrooms and ending up face-to-face with a copperhead. That's how he was inspired to invent this DIY mushroom hook.

Using a hook that Woody had given me as a model, it took me about 30 minutes of trial and error to make one to match his. After working out a system, it took only about 10 minutes to make subsequent hooks. Granted, not everyone has the tools or the interest in making even a low-tech tool like this. It may be a good opportunity for the handiest members of a mushroom club to make and sell them as a fund-raiser for the club. Or a self-employed mushroom hunter may want to offer them for sale to the public. I sell them at my foraging classes. And of course, I thank the innovative Captain Woody every time I do that.

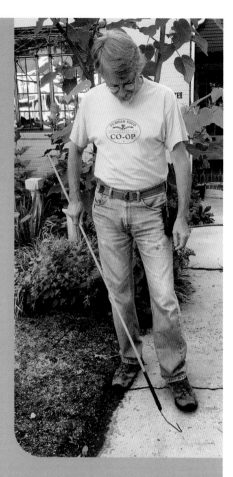

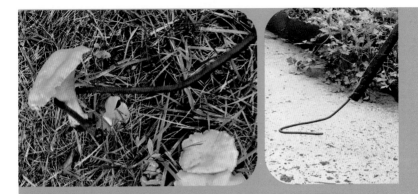

PARTS

- A 4- to 5-foot length of round fiberglass rod about ¼ to ½ inch thick. Some hardware stores sell them as posts for an electric fence.

- A 15-inch length of #9 tie wire. Also from hardware stores. When it's long it's limber, when it's short it's stiff.

- Duct tape.

- Optional: bright colored tape or paint for the handle, so you don't lose it in the woods.

TOOLS

- Tape measure.

- Speed square or some other way to determine angles.

- Handsaw, to cut fiberglass to length, if needed.

- Bolt cutters, to cut wire to length.

- Vice grips (or as we professionals call them, "the wrong tool for every job"), to bend wire into shape. Pliers will work, too.

- Hammer, to modify angle of the bent wire.

1 Wipe the light coating of oil off the wire and cut it to length (cut the fiberglass rod, too, if need be).

2 Use the vice grips to bend the wire double, 3 inches from its end.

3 The apex of the bend will be U-shaped. Rest it on a hard surface. Tap it with the hammer to get the bend into a V-shape. The V-shape is critical!

4 Then, with the vice grips, ease the wire back out to a 30-degree angle. That's your picker. If held parallel to the ground, it's at the correct angle for snagging a soilborne mushroom and holding the stalk securely.

5 About 5 inches from the apex of the V, with the V parallel to the ground, bend the straight end of the wire upward to form a 140-degree angle. You may need to adjust this angle a bit as you use it, to account for your height.

6 Tear off a 3-inch strip of duct tape to secure the straight end of the wire to the fiberglass rod.

7 Continue wrapping 3-inch lengths of tape around the wire and rod until you cover the entire wire. Make sure the tape is snug as you go.

8 Test-drive the mushroom picker with any soilborne mushrooms: Chanterelles, Morels, Milk Caps, Blewits, boletes, and so on. You may need to adjust the 140-degree angle a bit to get the V parallel to the ground. You may need to adjust the V itself until it holds a mushroom well.

9 Pull the hook horizontally to break the stem at the soil line. Pulling vertically will remove only the cap. Then celebrate like a sailor on shore leave.

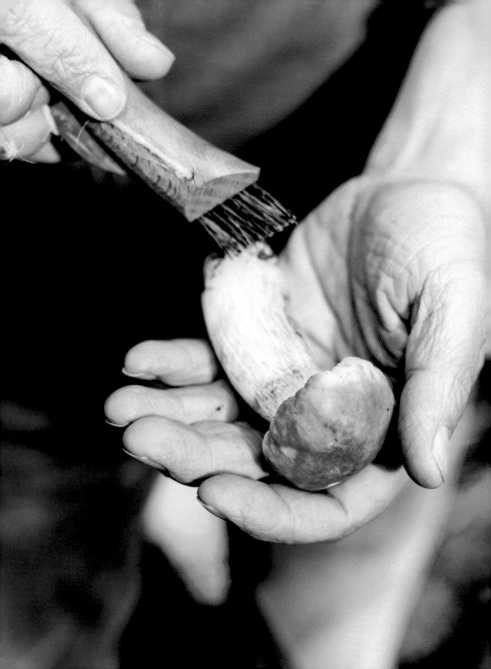

CHAPTER 7

Growing as a
MUSHROOM HUNTER

We all want to be eating tasty, nutrient-dense
foods, enjoying the fresh air,
and using our bodies in a balanced way.
Our ancestors coevolved with the fungi, plants,
and animals they hunted and gathered.
And we can coevolve, too. Here's how.

SOME FIRST STEPS

Learn about forays by finding and joining local foraging groups on Facebook or Meetup. Some people on these sites may also answer questions from novices. If you post photos of mushrooms you don't know, make them good photos. Show the top, bottom, and side of the mushroom. And if there any belowground parts, show them, too.

Get one or two field guides that cover your region. Actually, the best field guide for foraging will be one with two legs rather than two covers, but books can help reinforce what you learn. Also acquire some of the basic tools of the trade outlined in Chapter 6.

Now head outdoors!

CAN YOU FORAGE WHEN TRAVELING?

Some of my best dinner-party stories come from meeting foragers when we are traveling: eating wild food in Central Park in Manhattan; meeting an Italian forager who also had a wood-fired bread oven in his house; finding wild food in beach dunes with a photographer in South Carolina.

I find them by tasking Dr. Google with this search: "my destination" and "forager." Two-thirds of the time, some forager's website comes up and I can sign up for one of their classes or arrange a private tour. The rest of the time I find a reference to someone in an article or find someone who runs some other outdoor business. Either way, that gives me enough information to chase down an experienced forager.

If you do this, you'll realize two things. First, that foray was a highlight of your trip. Second, that it was probably also one of the least expensive things you did on your trip. In my experience, many self-employed people don't charge what their skill level is worth. If you feel that this is the case and you had a great experience, don't be afraid to give them a big tip if you're not poor. Fifty percent is not too much if you feel like the price was modest and the experience fantastic. By the time you're the one telling the best story at a dinner party, you will have forgotten how much you paid anyway.

HOW TO LEAD YOUR OWN FORAYS

You don't have to be a professional forager to lead a foray, and I wish more amateurs would do so. If there isn't an expert leading forays in your region, there's nothing stopping you from organizing one yourself. Many of the people who show up will know a few mushrooms and they can share their knowledge; you can fill in each other's gaps. It will also encourage you to step up your game of using your ID books to uncover the secret identities of mushrooms.

Use a Facebook or Meetup foraging group to announce when, where, and how long you want to forage. However many people show up is the right number, so don't feel bad if few people take you up on it. At least you are getting out in the woods.

Some public lands don't allow harvesting of mushrooms for sale or eating, so bear that in mind and choose a location where you know it's okay to harvest. Set a time for everyone to return to the parking lot, as folks may go separate routes in the woods. Spread a dark fabric on the ground on which people can lay the mushrooms they've gathered. Some names will be known and others will have to be looked up in books. Remind people to never eat anything that hasn't been identified with 100 percent certainty, then head off for beers. Or whatever. And since even a bad day of foraging is still a great day being outdoors, make plans to do it again.

SELLING MUSHROOMS

On occasion I make good money harvesting feral fungi for tattooed chefs. It would be tempting to try to make a full-time living from foraging. I know some people who do that, but I don't take it that far; if the rain clouds get shy, harvests will, too. But for the self-employed and semiretired, seasonal foraging can fill your basket with high-dollar food, outdoor fun, and quick cash.

Prices? For prime condition mushrooms, chefs are paying about as much per pound as you'd pay for New York strip steak or even filet mignon. Once I offered to sell Hen of the Woods to a chef and expected him to counter with a lower price. Instead he asked if I would accept some of my pay in gift cards to his restaurant at a higher price per pound; this spread out his costs and boosted my pay.

If you're lucky enough to find plenty to sell, you may want to follow my lead and engage in what I call "forager theater." Normally vendors are expected to come to the kitchen door at the back of the building; I did that when I was selling my organic tomatoes decades ago. But I've been getting away with flowing right through the front door and dining room (at a slow time, like between lunch and dinner) with edible fungi piled high in a shallow cardboard box, so diners can see them. I make sure everyone showing any curiosity gets a good look, and I answer their questions as I make my way back to the kitchen. Diners who see an actual forager with an exotic, wild mushroom will come back when it's on the menu.

No chef has complained about my delivery technique.

Even if I never did make a dime, I'd still be foraging. Flavors aside, it's a sensation I can't buy. Finding and eating wild mushrooms triggers a quiet hum in my chest that tells me I'm a part of nature, not just a spectator.

GETTING CERTIFIED TO SELL WILD MUSHROOMS

There are states where it's illegal to sell foraged mushrooms. Some of these laws stem from the time when the powers that be wanted to keep college kids from tripping on psylocibin mushrooms. Legislators wanted to make the shrooms illegal, but the police asked how they would know which mushrooms were which. So they made all wild mushrooms illegal.

That was the state of things in much of the United States until people like Tradd Cotter in South Carolina decided to overcome that hurdle. By testing foragers' knowledge, Tradd has helped them get certified to sell wild mushrooms. Tradd has worked with public health staff in several states to set up his classes and certification.

So if you're considering selling wild mushrooms to restaurants or at the farmers' market, you should first check with your county or state health department to find out if you need certification.

Tradd's business—Mushroom Mountain—provides certification in seven East Coast states: Georgia, South Carolina, North Carolina, Virginia, Pennsylvania, New York, and Rhode Island, so check there first for details.

Resources

References

White Paper on Strategies to Reduce Risks and Expand Appreciation of Foraged Wild Mushrooms
https://namyco.org/docs/EdiblePoisonousReport20170914.pdf

"Edible Mushroom-Related Poisoning: A Study on Circumstances of Mushroom Collection, Transport, and Storage"
https://journals.sagepub.com/doi/full/10.1177/0960327114557901

Books and Magazines for Mushroom Hunters

To reinforce your newfound knowledge, pick up a brace of books. A regional guidebook to mushrooms is the best place to start, and back that up with these great books.

MUSHROOM ID

Alaska's Mushrooms by Harriette Parker

All That the Rain Promises and More . . . by David Arora

Amanitas of North America by Britt A. Bunyard and Jay Justice

Backyard Foraging by Ellen Zachos

The Book of Fungi by Peter Roberts and Shelley Evans

The Complete Mushroom Hunter by Gary Lincoff

Edible and Medicinal Mushrooms of New England and Eastern Canada by David L. Spahr

The Essential Guide to Rocky Mountain Mushrooms by Habitat by Cathy L. Cripps, Vera S. Evenson, and Michael Kuo

Fascinating Fungi of the North Woods by Cora Mollen and Larry Weber

A Field Guide to Mushrooms of the Carolinas by Alan E. Bessette, Arleen R. Bessette, and Michael W. Hopping

Mushrooms Demystified by David Arora

Mushrooms of the Southeast by Todd F. Elliott and Steven L. Stephenson

North American Boletes by Alan E. Bessette, William C. Roody, and Arleen R. Bessette

100 Edible Mushrooms by Michael Kuo

The Scout's Guide to Wild Edibles by Mike Krebill

Toxic and Hallucinogenic Mushroom Poisoning by Gary Lincoff and D. H. Mitchell, MD

THE FORAGING LIFE

Beatrix Potter by Linda Lear

Eating Wildly by Ava Chin

Fat of the Land by Langdon Cook

The Mushroom Hunters by Langdon Cook

Stalking the Wild Asparagus by Euell Gibbons

The Way Through the Woods by Long Litt Woon

ESSAYS AND USEFUL TIPS ABOUT FORAGING

Fungipedia: A Brief Compendium of Mushroom Lore by Lawrence Millman

Mushroom by Nicholas P. Money

Mycophilia: Revelations from the Weird World of Mushrooms by Eugenia Bone

COOKBOOKS

The Complete Mushroom Book: The Quiet Hunt by Antonio Carluccio

The Mushroom Hunter's Kitchen: Reimagining Comfort Food with a Chef Forager by Chad Hyatt

The Wild Vegan Cookbook by "Wildman" Steve Brill

CULTIVATION

Organic Mushroom Farming and Mycoremediation by Tradd Cotter

QUARTERLY MAGAZINES

Fungi Magazine
www.fungimag.com

Mushroom: The Journal of Wild Mushrooming
www.mushroomthejournal.com

Helpful Websites

The Bolete Filter
https://boletes.wpamushroom
club.org
The Western Pennsylvania Mushroom club maintains a very helpful rogue's gallery of boletes they call the Bolete Filter.

MushroomExpert.com
www.mushroomexpert.com
If your smartphone has reception when you're in the woods, this is a helpful site for keying out a mystery mushroom. If you are 99 percent or less certain about ID, don't eat the mushroom.

LINKS TO RECIPES

Medicinal Chaga with Hot Chocolate
www.youtube.com
/watch?v=4akg8BpJSxM
Courtesy of Adam Haritan of Learn Your Land

Techniques for Preparing Chicken of the Woods

http://ledameredith.com/chicken-of-the-woods-mushroom-and-what-to-do-with-old-chickens

Leda Meredith has authored foraging books for the Northeast. This link leads you to her clever technique for flavoring food with medicinal Turkey Tail, as well as her techniques for preparing Chicken of the Woods, both in its prime and even when it has grown too tough for common cooking techniques.

Stuffings and Bread Pudding

https://backyardforager.com/wild-mushroom-stuffing-recipe

https://backyardforager.com/asparagus-mushroom-bread-pudding

Ellen Zachos writes books on foraging in your own yard and on making cocktails with wild ingredients.

Asian-Inspired Oysters

http://langdoncook.com/2019/04/23/stir-fried-oyster-mushrooms-with-chicken

Langdon Cook is an author and forager in the Pacific Northwest.

Lion's Mane Croquettes and Beefsteak Sashimi

https://mushroommountain.com/cooking-with-wild-mushrooms

Olga Cotter is a southern forager and co-owner (with her husband Tradd Cotter) of Mushroom Mountain, a world-class fungi research facility.

Pickled Mushrooms

instagram.com/p/B3hVB8VpLDR
instagram.com/p/B25MzauJ_z6

Pascal Baudar forages in southern California and has written books on cooking, brewing, and fermenting with foraged ingredients.

Hen of the Woods Jerky

http://the3foragers.blogspot.com/2018/09/the-original-mushroom-jerky-hen-of.html

Shrimp Mocktail

www.wildmanstevebrill.com/mushroom-recipes

"Wildman" Steve Brill was arrested for foraging in Central Park, subsequently becoming the inspiration for a character on *Seinfeld*. He's written books on foraging with kids, medicinal mushrooms, and vegan cooking with wild ingredients, among others. His website contains nearly 50 mushroom recipes.

Hedgehog Conserve

https://foragerchef.com/hedgehog-mushrooms

Alan Bergo, the forager chef, posts regularly on Instagram (@foragerchef) and has a wealth of mushroom recipes and cooking techniques on his website.

Turkey Tail Tea

www.organifishop.com/blogs/news/3-ways-to-make-turkey-tail-tea

These folks offer three ways to make Turkey Tail tea.

OTHER WAYS TO USE MUSHROOMS

How to Start a Fire with Tinder Conk

http://paulkirtley.co.uk/2011/easy-way-to-use-fomes-fomentarius-as-tinder

Courtesy of Paul Kirtley, a top-ranked bushcraft blogger.

Medicinal Uses for Reishi

https://redmoonherbs.com/blogs/womens-health-and-herbal-medicine/how-to-get-the-most-medicine-out-of-your-reishi-mushrooms

Courtesy of the lovely folks at Red Moon Herbs.

Acknowledgments

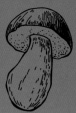

Many thanks to the cheerful, effective staff of Storey for some of the best professional experiences of my life, including Carleen Madigan, Carolyn Eckert, Jennifer Jepson Smith, Alee Moncy, Anastasia Whalen, Jennifer Travis, Melinda Slaving, and Tina Parent.

Many thanks to Tradd and Olga Cotter for opening the doors of perception to all those interested in Hens, Chickens, and Lion's Manes spilling out of trees.

Grazie mille to Severino for keeping his eye on me while on Mount Amiata.

Tip of the hat to Alan Muskat of No Taste Like Home for your fungal rap and fine thoughts.

A hearty "can't wait till next time" to Parker Veitch for those snowmobile-trail hikes.

And a Lowcountry shout-out to Woody Collins for driving me through the woods in a VW Beetle and for many other fine adventures in foraging, eating, and story swapping.

Last, I apologize for leaving anyone out, I but want to acknowledge (in no particular order) the guidance of other foragers who've generously shared their time and knowledge with me: "Wildman" Steve Brill, Ellen Zachos, Mike Krebill, Doug Elliott, Gumby Montgomery, Sam and Melissa Thayer, Leda Meredith, Pascal Baudar, Langdon Cook, John Doughty, Russ Cohen, Kerry Hardy, Nan Chase, Marie Viljoen, Susan Hitchcock, John Kallas, David Spahr, Andrew Cebulka, Adam Haritan, Britt Bunyard, Leon Shernoff, Marc Williams, Anna McHugh, Randy Faulkner, Gregory Bonito, Mike Hopping, Green Deane, Will Endres, Adolpho Rosati, and Maurizio Gioli.

Metric Conversion Charts

Unless you have finely calibrated measuring equipment, conversions between US and metric measurements will be somewhat inexact. It's important to convert the measurements for all of the ingredients in a recipe or project to maintain the same proportions as the original.

WEIGHT

TO CONVERT	TO	MULTIPLY
ounces	grams	ounces by 28.35
pounds	grams	pounds by 453.5
pounds	kilograms	pounds by 0.45

VOLUME

TO CONVERT	TO	MULTIPLY
teaspoons	milliliters	teaspoons by 4.93
tablespoons	milliliters	tablespoons by 14.79
fluid ounces	milliliters	fluid ounces by 29.57
cups	milliliters	cups by 236.59
cups	liters	cups by 0.24
pints	milliliters	pints by 473.18
pints	liters	pints by 0.473
quarts	milliliters	quarts by 946.36
quarts	liters	quarts by 0.946
gallons	liters	gallons by 3.785

TEMPERATURE

TO CONVERT	TO	
Fahrenheit	Celsius	subtract 32 from Fahrenheit temperature, multiply by 5, then divide by 9

LENGTH

TO CONVERT	TO	MULTIPLY
inches	millimeters	inches by 25.4
inches	centimeters	inches by 2.54
inches	meters	inches by 0.0254
feet	meters	feet by 0.3048
feet	kilometers	feet by 0.0003048
yards	centimeters	yards by 91.44
yards	meters	yards by 0.9144
yards	kilometers	yards by 0.0009144
miles	meters	miles by 1,609.344
miles	kilometers	miles by 1.609344

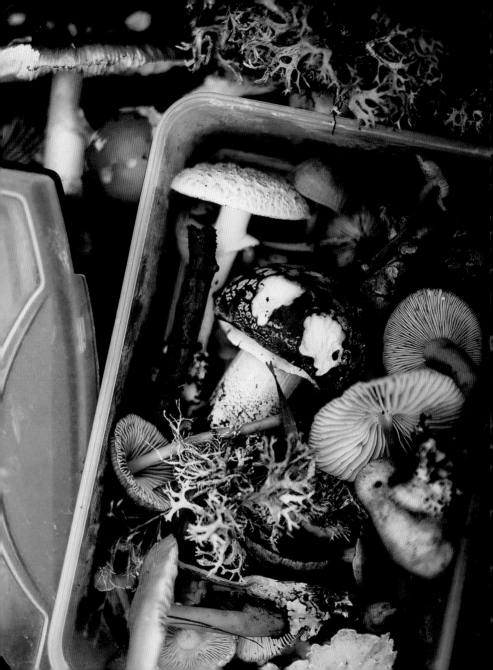

Index

Page numbers in *italic* indicate images and **bold** indicate tables.

Interior Photography Credits

Interior photography by © 2008 Alan Cressler/Wikimedia Commons/CC BY-SA 3.0, 69; © 2009 Dan Molter (shroomydan)/Wikimedia Commons/CC BY-SA 3.0, 72; © 2009 Dan Molter (shroomydan)/Mushroom Observer/Wikimedia Commons/CC BY-SA 3.0/Wikimedia Commons, 169; © 2009 Ron Pastorino (Ronpast)/Wikimedia Commons/CC BY-SA 3.0, 144 t.; © 2013 Dr. Lorne Stobbs (Stobbsl)/Mushroom Observer/Wikimedia Commons/CC BY-SA 3.0, 162; © Akela - from alp to alp/Stocksy, 228; © Aleksandr Ugorenkov/stock.adobe.com, 143 l.; © Alexander Kurlovich/stock.adobe.com, 96 & 205 b.; © Alika/stock.adobe.com, 55 t.; © am13photo/stock.adobe.com, 133 t. & 136; © Amelia Martin/Alamy Stock Photo, 116; © Amy Buxton/stock.adobe.com, 174 t.r.; © Andrea Obzerova/Alamy Stock Photo, 27 r.; Annie Spratt/Unsplash, 5 & 248; © arihen/stock.adobe.com, 190 b.; © Arpad/stock.adobe.com, 81; © arska n/stock.adobe.com, 207; © Artenex/stock.adobe.com, 133 b.; © Arterra Picture Library/Alamy Stock Photo, 138 t.; Atik Sulianami/Unsplash, 12; © Barbora Batokova/stock.adobe.com, 110, 111 b.l., 120 t., 160; © Barry/stock.adobe.com, 180 & 182; © Beginner photographer/iStock.com, 51; © bobleccinum/stock.adobe.com, 196; © Bogdan Mihai/stock.adobe.com, 24; © Cameron Zegers/Stocksy, 6 & 34; Carolyn Eckert © Storey Publishing LLC, 23; © Chris Zielecki/Stocksy, 1; © Cosma Andrei/Stocksy, 15; © Darina Kopcok/Stocksy, 214; © David Cobb/Alamy Stock Photo, 53 b.; © Denis Gavrilov/stock.adobe.com, 66; © Denis/stock.adobe.com, 49 l.; © dm/stock.adobe.com, 193; ekamelev/Unsplash, 36; © Emma/stock.adobe.com, 122; © Empire331/Dreamstime.com, 174 b.r.; © Erika Bailey, 30 b.; © fotocof/stock.adobe.com, 124 b.; © Frank Hecker/Alamy Stock Photo, 128 l.; © Frank Hyman, 105, 201, 231, 232; © Gabi Wolf/Alamy Stock Photo, 208 l.; © Giulio/stock.adobe.com, 32; © Hakan Soderholm/Alamy Stock Photo, 68; © HandmadePictures/stock.adobe.com, 218; © hekakoskinen/iStock.com, 73 & 74; © Henri Koskinen/Alamy Stock Photo, 53 t.; © Henri Koskinen/stock.adobe.com, 112 b., 128 r., 188; © Henrik Larsson/stock.adobe.com, 172; © Horst Könemund/stock.adobe.com, 202 t.r.; © Igor Kramar/stock.adobe.com, 138 m. & b., 147, 157, 189, 205 t.; © imageBROKER/Alamy Stock Photo, 108; © Ina Peters/Stocksy, 8, 222, 234; © Ionescu Bogdan/stock.adobe.com, 28 b., 29, 86, 119, 158, 194 r.; © Ivan/stock.adobe.com, 59, 141, 190 t.l.; © Iwona/stock.adobe.com, 106; © Jack Barr/Alamy Stock Photo, 208 r.; © James/stock.adobe.com, 184 & 185; © Jaroslav Machacek/stock.adobe.com, 76, 84, 127, 134 l., 148 l.; © Jarrod Erbe/Shutterstock.

LEARN MORE ABOUT WILD FOODS
with these other Storey books

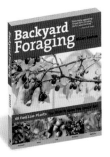

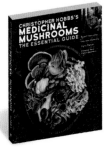

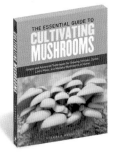

BACKYARD FORAGING
by Ellen Zachos
Food grows everywhere! Photographic profiles of 70 edible weeds, flowers, and other plants, along with expert advice on safety and sustainability, help you discover what your neighborhood has to offer.

CHRISTOPHER HOBBS'S MEDICINAL MUSHROOMS: THE ESSENTIAL GUIDE
An herbalist and renowned mushroom expert introduces you to the varieties most widely used for medicinal purposes. Learn about their health benefits, the science behind their therapeutic power, and how to make your own mushroom medicines.

THE ESSENTIAL GUIDE TO CULTIVATING MUSHROOMS
by Stephen Russell
With clear instructions and step-by-step photographs, this straightforward guide shows you how to successfully grow mushrooms at home.